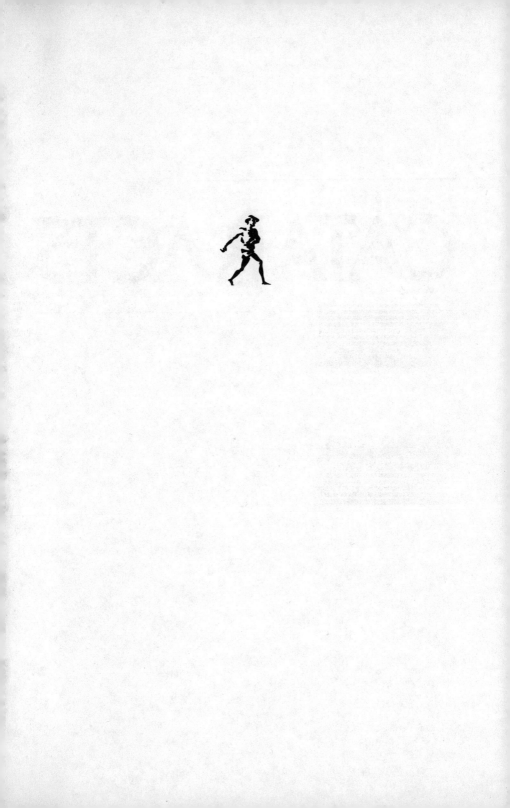

CATARACTS

The Complete Guide
-From Diagnosis to Recovery-
For Patients and Families

Julius Shulman, M.D.

Illustrations by Neil O. Hardy

SIMON AND SCHUSTER • NEW YORK

Published by Simon and Schuster
A Division of Simon & Schuster, Inc.
Simon & Schuster Building
Rockefeller Center
1230 Avenue of the Americas
New York, New York 10020
SIMON AND SCHUSTER and colophon are registered trademarks of
Simon & Schuster, Inc.
Designed by Eve Kirch
Manufactured in the United States of America

1   3   5   7   9   10   8   6   4   2

Library of Congress Cataloging in Publication Data

Shulman, Julius, date.
Cataracts: the complete guide—from diagnosis to
recovery—for patients and families.
Includes index.
1. Cataract.   I. Title.
RE451.S365   1984   617.7′42   83-19145

ISBN 0–671–46917–7

Acknowledgments

It is with immense gratitude and appreciation that I thank Barbara Bannon, whose guidance and support were a catalyst for this book. My friend, Jethro Lieberman, a.k.a. W. M., abetted this undertaking and has only himself to blame. Special thanks goes to my editor, Bob Bender, whose tactful hints and suggestions were invaluable. Gloria J. Bennett typed superbly, tirelessly and enthusiastically and I cannot thank her enough. Dr. Robert Coles and my brothers, Howie and Marty, know their role in all this and I will be forever in their debt. Lastly I want to thank my wife, Shelli, whose encouragement was frequent, earnest and deeply appreciated.

To my wife, Shelli,
children, Ilana, Lauren, Michael;
and to my father and to my mother, who,
perhaps, can somehow read this.

Contents

Preface

If you are reading this book, chances are that you or someone close to you has been told you have a cataract. Perhaps you are contemplating cataract surgery or have had an operation already. Since a half million cataract operations are performed each year in the United States alone, you are in good company. This book will help you understand the nature of cataracts and cataract surgery—whether or not to have an operation and if so, what type. The technological revolution in eye surgery has made it difficult for the layperson to understand the many types of cataract surgery and arrive at an intelligent and correct decision. If you have already had surgery this book should answer many of your questions that may have been left unresolved. It will also aid you in getting through those first few postoperative weeks, when your sight

11

may constantly change, your eye may be a source of anxiety and apprehension and things may actually seem worse before they get better. Rest assured though. The success rate for cataract surgery is almost 95 percent, so the chances are excellent that you will fully regain your sight.

1

What Is a Cataract ?

"Your vision is blurred because you have cataracts."

This diagnosis is made by ophthalmologists throughout the world hundreds of times every day. Cataracts
are one of the most common afflictions known. In its
early stages a cataract is not a disease at all, but a normal part of aging. It is one of the leading causes of
blindness in the United States, and although it is more
common as you get older, it can even be present at
birth. If we live long enough, almost all of us will develop cataracts.

A cataract is a loss of transparency, or clouding, of
the normally clear lens of the eye. In order to see
sharply and clearly, light must pass into your eye
through a crystal-clear lens, just as a sharply focused
picture depends on light passing through a clear camera lens. As you get older chemical changes occur in
the human lens that render it less transparent. The loss

13

of transparency may be so mild as to hardly affect vision, or be so severe that no shapes or movements are seen, only light and dark. When the lens gets cloudy enough to obstruct vision to any significant degree, it is called a cataract.

The origin of the word "cataract" is fascinating though somewhat obscure, stemming from misconceptions during Greek and Roman times that cataracts were evil liquids that flowed into the eye. A papyrus dating to 1500 B.C. describes what was probably a cataract under the term "the mounting of water in the eye." The Greeks used the words *hypochyma* and *hypochysis,* meaning "water underneath," while the Romans used the Latin term *suffusis* to describe a cataract as a suffusion, or overspreading. During the Middle Ages the Arabs translated the term for cataract into an Arabic word meaning "black water." At the end of the Middle Ages the Arabic for "black water" was translated back into Latin as the word *cataracta*—a waterfall. The Latin cataracta became the English cataract.

Although cataracts were recognized more than 3,000 years ago, it took centuries for medicine to begin to understand the nature and causes of this malady. Learned scholars such as Leonardo da Vinci (1452–1519) and Andreas Vesalius (1514–1564) staunchly maintained that a cataract was an evil humor or phlegm which covered and clouded the front of the lens, rather than a disease of the lens itself.

Credit goes to Warner Rolfink (1599–1673), an anatomy professor in Jena, Italy, for first publishing the true nature of a cataract. Professor Rolfink learned of the French surgeon François Quarre, who thought that a cataract was merely a clouded lens. By the gruesome task of dissecting the eyes of executed criminals (of which there were plenty), Rolfink confirmed his theory.

In order to understand what's going on inside the eye and how the lens turns cloudy, you have to bear with me as we learn more about the human lens. The next chapter describes the workings of the whole eye, but for now let's get a good foundation for understanding your cataract—we start with the lens.

The *lens* is a transparent organ about the size of a pea that sits just behind the *iris,* the colored part of your eye (*see Figure 1*). There are three parts to the lens: the *capsule,* the *nucleus* and the *cortex.* The capsule is a thin membrane which completely surrounds the lens much like the skin of a peach. When we are young the center of the lens, the nucleus, is soft, almost the consistency of custard. As we get older, into our fifties and sixties, the nucleus gets sclerotic, or hard, somewhat resembling the pit of a peach. The rest of the lens is made up of long, arching fibers, running from top to bottom, called the cortex. As we age the older fibers are pushed to the center of the lens and compacted, while the newer, looser fibers are near the outside. To switch analogies, the growth of

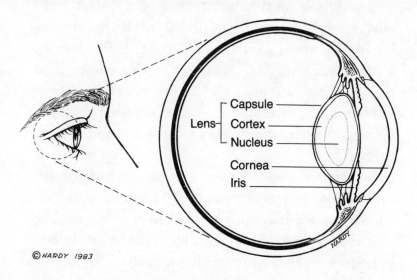

© HARDY 1983

Figure 1. The three parts of the lens with the cornea and the iris.

the lens resembles that of a tree—both continue to grow throughout life with the older part in the center and the newer on the outside.

The function of the lens is to refract, or bend, light rays to focus them to a clear image on the back of the eye. The lens, being somewhat elastic, will change shape to properly focus light, getting fatter for close objects, such as the type on this page, and thinner for distant objects, such as a street sign. Starting as early as age twenty, the lens slowly loses its elasticity, until at around age forty it cannot change shape enough to bring close objects into focus. Reading glasses will then be necessary to aid in focusing. The shape of the lens is automatically controlled by muscles that line the wall of the eye called *ciliary muscles.* The muscles encircle the lens like a headband and are connected to it by *zonules,* thin jellylike strands that hold the lens in place like suspenders. If it wasn't for the zonules, the lens would sink to the bottom of the eye like a pebble dropped into a glass of water. Although each zonule is weak by itself, the suspensory framework formed by thousands of them is amazingly strong.

The lens has the highest protein content of any organ in the body, 33 percent compared to 18 percent for muscle. You can cut a T-bone steak as thin as you possibly can and yet you will not be able to see through it, but the lens is easily transparent and yet has almost twice the protein content of steak. The reason for this miracle is the unique physical and chemical arrangement of the protein fibers in the lens, as opposed to the more variable arrangement of fibers in steak or any other nontransparent part of our body. If even a very small part of the lens gets cloudy enough to block rays of light, be it the central nucleus, the outer cortex, or the thin surrounding capsule, that part is called an opacity. If enough opacities form in the lens to affect vision, or if a general loss of transparency occurs, the end result is a cataractous lens—a cataract. A cataract is not a skin or a film over the eye, nor is it a growth or infection. It is merely a loss of transparency of the normally clear lens. The more cloudy the lens and the more it involves the center of the lens, the worse the vision.

To better understand cataracts, we ought to review how the eye works.

2

How the Eye Sees

A simple explanation of how the eye sees is that the eye does not do the seeing, the brain does. In fact the eye is really an extension of the brain and gathers information for processing much the same way a TV antenna gathers a signal for the television to convert into a picture. We will now examine each part of the eye in order to get a better understanding of the vision process.

If you look at your eye in a mirror, the most obvious feature is its color. This comes from a pigmented structure called the *iris* (*see Figure 2*). We are all born with lightly colored eyes, and if the iris becomes very pigmented we wind up with brown eyes. The less the pigment, the bluer your eyes will be. If you look a little more closely, you will see a black hole in the middle of the iris. This is the *pupil*, the opening

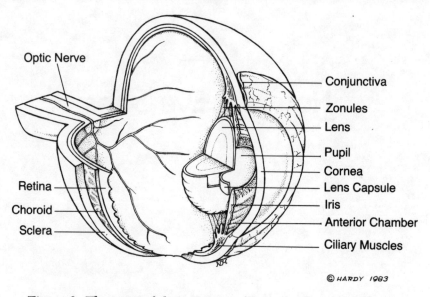

Optic Nerve

Conjunctiva

Zonules

Lens

Pupil

Cornea

Retina

Lens Capsule

Choroid

Iris

Sclera

Anterior Chamber

Ciliary Muscles

© HARDY 1983

Figure 2. The parts of the eye.

through which light travels into your eye. The pupil controls the amount of light that enters the eye, becoming smaller in bright light and larger in dim light. If you take a flashlight and shine it into your eye while looking at the pupil in a mirror, you will see the constant adjustment in pupil size as light hits your eye. What you probably cannot see is a sparkling-clear dome-shaped membrane which vaults over the front of the eye like a skylight on a roof. This is the *cornea*, and clear vision is as much dependent on a clear cornea as on a clear lens. When a foreign body hits your eye it invariably lands on the cornea, whose rich supply of pain fibers immediately announces its presence. The *sclera,* the white of the eye, surrounds the cornea and extends completely around the back of the eye. This forms a tough outer wall giving the eye strength and substance.

A thin membrane, the *conjunctiva,* covers the white of the eye and lines the inside of the lids. The conjunctiva has tiny blood vessels which can become enlarged with mild infection, allergy or pollution causing the eye to look bloodshot. Conjunctivitis, or pinkeye, results when this layer becomes infected.

Working together, the cornea, the pupil and the lens focus light onto the back of the eye, the *retina.* This is a thin, diaphanous membrane which lines the inside of the back of the eye. The retina, likened to the film in a camera, "takes" the picture, and the brain "develops" it. The retina sends the picture to the brain by way of a thick nerve in the back of the eye, the *optic nerve.* As illustrated in Figure 2, there is an inner layer of the eye, the retina, as well as an outer layer, the sclera. There is also a middle layer, the *choroid,* darkly pigmented, resembling the skin of a grape. In fact, another name for this is the uvea, which means "grape" in Latin. This grape skin, or uvea, forms the iris in the front of the eye and the choroid in the back of the eye. Most of the blood circulation which nourishes the eye travels in the choroid.

Two other parts of the eye deserve mention, since they make up the fluid portion of the eye. The space between the iris and cornea, called the *anterior chamber,* is filled with *aqueous,* a solution resembling spinal fluid. New aqueous is constantly being formed to replace aqueous which filters out of the eye. A blockage of this results in elevated pressure in the eye—glaucoma. Most of the inside cavity of the eye is filled with the *vitreous,* a jellylike material which gives the eye substance and volume.

Let's see what happens, from front to back, when a ray of light enters your eye. How is a painting transformed from a mixture of oils, pigments and canvas to a picture of color, texture, depth and warmth in your brain? Each part of the eye plays a role.

Light bouncing off a painting or a tree or a book will first hit your cornea, the clear dome-shaped front part of your eye. The image will now be about 60 percent focused as the rays of light are bent (refracted) by the cornea. Light then passes through the pupil and enters the lens, which bends the rays of light another 40 percent. This should result, in the ideal situation, in an image focused to a sharp point on the retina.

Only when light is focused to a sharp point will the image be clear. The light acts like an electric shock through the ten layers of cells in the retina and stimulates them to send their message to the brain. Most of the light is focused on an area of the retina called the *macula,* and this is where vision is the sharpest and clearest. It is this "central vision" which allows us to read, watch a movie or drive a car. The rest of the retina gives peripheral, or side, vision, also important in driving a car and generally getting around. Without peripheral vision we would be left with only "tunnel vision" and would continuously walk into things in our path. The cells in the macula which enable us to see sharp detail are called *cones,* as opposed to the *rods* in the remainder of the retina which give peripheral vision. The cones are mostly active in vision during daylight and also supply us with color vision. There are cones for red, green and blue, and how we appreciate the hundreds of colors in our environment via cells for only the three primary colors is truly amazing and still not completely understood.

If the light rays were always focused to a sharp point on the retina, we would never need glasses. We need glasses, or have a refractive error, when this point of focus falls in front of the retina, as in myopia (nearsightedness), or behind the retina, as in hyperopia (farsightedness). In spite of its complexity, the retina merely sends to the brain whatever image it receives, clear or blurred. Glasses will correct the refractive error and clear up the blurred image by focusing the rays of light on the retina. Astigmatism, from the Greek *a,* meaning "without," and *stigma,* meaning "point," results when the image is not focused to a point at all, usually because of an irregularly shaped cornea. Glasses for astigmatism first have to bend the light rays to a point, whether in front or in back of the retina, and then bring this point to a sharp focus on the retina itself.

Vision is measured using the familiar Snellen chart which has lines of increasingly smaller numbers. Each line of the chart corresponds to a different level of vision, such as 20/400, 20/100, 20/70, 20/40 and 20/20, which is somewhat arbitrarily designated as "normal." The vision of each eye is expressed as a fraction: the top number represents the testing distance from the chart, and the bottom number the distance from the chart at which a normal eye could see. If while standing 20 feet from the chart, your right eye, for example, can see only the larger numbers such as the 85 comprising the 20/200 line, the vision in your right eye would be designated 20/200 (*see Figure 3*). (A normal eye would be able to see this from 200 feet away.) If one eye sees 20/20 and the other eye, the one with the cataract, sees 20/100, the total vision of the person would still be 20/20. This is a very important point for pa-

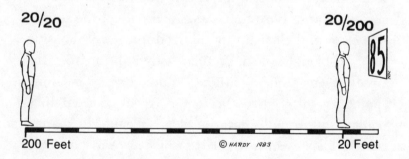

Figure 3. The eye chart. If a person must stand at a 20-foot distance to see the "85" seen by a person with normal vision at 200 feet, that person is said to have 20/200 vision.

tients with a cataract in one eye and a normal, clear lens in the other eye. A cataract does not have to be removed just because it's there. We'll learn more about that in Chapter 7.

Now that we know what a cataract is, and how the normal eye sees, let's get to what brings you to the eye doctor in the first place—the symptoms of a cataract.

3

Symptoms of a Cataract

"I'm not sure I'm seeing as I used to. I keep thinking my glasses are dirty and things just don't seem right."

"When I look at TV I get a double image. I see two televisions instead of one!"

"I'm getting better in my old age. I don't need my reading glasses anymore!"

"What's the matter with my doctor? I got three pairs of glasses in the last six months! I'm still not seeing right!"

"Bright lights make me so blurred I can't even cross the street on a sunny day. I don't see how it's possible but I see better on a cloudy day!"

"Colors don't seem as bright as they used to—everything seems kind of yellow, like there's a film over my eye."

All these statements suggest the presence of cataracts. Let's examine them one by one.

The first complaint is the most common symptom of a cataract: You are not seeing as well as you did in the past. This can often be so subtle as to confuse patient and doctor alike. It starts as a subjective change, a slight inkling, a nagging feeling that something is wrong with your sight. Initially there may be no supporting objective findings—you may still be 20/20—but that clock across the street does not seem as clear as it was six months ago. You keep thinking your glasses are dirty, your eyes are tired. A typical visit to your ophthalmologist may contain the following:

PATIENT: Doctor, something is wrong, I'm not seeing right.

DOCTOR: Well, I checked your vision and it's still 20/20, or just about. And you don't need any change in glasses; that won't help. I do detect some very early changes in the lens of your eyes, but you are seventy-three years old and this is probably normal aging rather than true cataracts. The rest of your eye examination is perfectly normal, so let me check you again in about six months. Please call me if anything develops before that.

Suppose this patient is an accountant, and is quite aware of slight changes in his vision. Another patient might have been less sensitive to these changes or subconsciously denied them as many of us do with anxiety-producing symptoms. In that case the visit may have taken place quite a few months later and been entirely different:

PATIENT: Doctor, something is wrong, I'm not seeing right.

DOCTOR: I'm surprised you've gone this long with the vision the way it is. The vision in your right eye has dropped from 20/20 to 20/40 and your left eye is only seeing 20/70. You definitely have incipient cataracts.

Each patient reacted differently to his symptoms, one being sensitive to the slight change in vision and the other waiting until the diminished vision was more noticeable.

Seeing double is caused by a cataract that is not uniformly dense or opaque. One part of the lens may have more opacities than another, causing rays of light, such as from a TV screen, to split into two or even three different parts. This is especially true of a small cataract in the nucleus, the central hard part of the lens. Here's an easy test to determine if double vision is from a cataract: cover the good eye and see if the double vision disappears. If it does, the cataract is not causing double vision and most likely the eye muscles are at fault, causing your eyes to be misaligned.

The newly acquired ability to read without glasses is another common symptom of cataracts, and the understandable enthusiasm for this "second sight" belies a developing cataract. The explanation lies in the part of the lens first affected by the cataractous process. As we learned in Chapter 2, the lens is divided into three parts—an outer capsule, an inner central nucleus and the fibers in between, the cortex. If the cataract starts in the central nuclear area, the nucleus will become hard or sclerotic, the same way cholesterol deposits in arteries cause hardening of the arteries, or arteriosclerosis. This causes the lens to get fatter and optically stronger, so that light will be focused in front of the retina. The net effect on the eye is that it becomes nearsighted. This nearsightedness can enable you to read without glasses, and may be the only clue to a developing cataract. In fact the lens at this stage may not look cataractous at all but may appear completely normal.

Nearsightedness from a developing cataract also explains the necessity for frequent changes of glasses. As you become more and more nearsighted, the glasses must keep pace with the changes in your eye. While this may be a nuisance, you should realize how fortunate you are in being able to maintain your usual level of vision in spite of changes in glasses. As the cataract matures, however, glasses will no longer maintain your sight and surgery will eventually be necessary.

Poor vision in bright light may seem paradoxical at first. If a cataract cuts down on the light entering the eye, shouldn't more light help? The answer depends on the type of cataract and which part of the lens is affected. When most of the opacity in the lens is concentrated in the center of the lens, especially on the back, or posterior surface, it will have its greatest impact when the pupil, or opening into the eye, is small. The brighter the light, the smaller the pupil and the greater effect the cataract may have in blocking vision. This may be quite incapacitating to a patient with such a cataract, technically called a posterior subcapsular cataract, as anything other than a cloudy day may markedly reduce visual acuity. This may not even be apparent in the ophthalmologist's office, because most of the time the room is fairly dark when vision is tested. Should your ophthalmologist detect a posterior subcapsular cataract, your vision should be retested with the room lights on; this will give a more realistic assessment of your diminished eyesight. Drops which open or dilate the pupil may allow light to be focused around the cataract and may improve vision dramatically. I can think of several patients who were helped with this treatment and were able to forestall surgery for over a year. Unfortunately, this type of cataract is often associated with long-term use of cortisone, for such diseases as arthritis, asthma and gastrointestinal diseases.

The last symptom of a cataract, a change in color vision, is a subtle alteration in the quality of your vision, which may be overshadowed by more noticeable alterations in the clarity of your vision. As the cataract progresses, the nucleus becomes more and more yellow. In becoming yellower the cataract absorbs wavelengths of first violet and then blue light, effectively reducing those colors and making the environment appear yellowish. The opposite effect often occurs immediately after cataract surgery, when a flood of blue and violet light enters the eye and everything looks blue.

The underlying theme that runs through all the symptoms of a cataract is that your eyesight is getting worse. The change is usually quite gradual and painless and occurs over months and years. Lights may cause glare, colors may look yellow, you may sense a film over your eyes, but the dominant problem is that you just can't see as well as you used to. If a cataract develops in only one eye and that is your nondominant eye, you may not even know it is there until the vision in that eye is surprisingly poor. To find your dominant eye, bring together the tip of your thumb and forefinger into an "O," about six inches from your face. It is important to keep both eyes open. Focus on an object across the room so that it is in the middle of the "O." Closing one eye and then the other will tell you which eye is dominant. If you close your left eye and the object is still in the center of the "O," then your right eye was the "sighting" eye and is the dominant one and vice versa. If a choice were possible, it would be better to have a cataract in your nondominant eye, because good vision in your dominant eye will feel more comfortable and natural. An ophthalmologist I know developed a cataract in his dominant, right eye, but deferred surgery for a while because his left eye was still 20/20. Only after cataract surgery restored 20/20 vision to his dominant eye did he really feel he could see again.

What causes cataracts to develop? We'll discuss in the next chapter some of the reasons cataracts are so common.

4

What Causes Cataracts?

Some loss of transparency of the lens will happen to all of us if we live long enough, and the resulting change in the lens, if significant, is called a *senile cataract*. This term comes from the Latin word for "old" and has nothing to do with mental faculties or behavior. Age is the major predisposing cause of cataracts, and cataracts are part of the price paid for increasing longevity. In much the same way our hair will gray, our hearing diminish and our joints develop arthritis.

Of the two million people in the United States with visually disabling cataracts, well over 90 percent have senile cataracts. The majority of people in their seventies and eighties show some mild cataractous changes, but since these changes generally do not significantly affect vision they would not be termed a true cataract but just normal changes in the lens due to age. The lens may be a little yellow or cloudy, and vision may be somewhat reduced by one or two lines on the eye chart. This change in vision need not and probably will not interfere with reading, driving, television and any other daily activity.

A study done in 1968 in the United States showed that more than 80 percent of people over age sixty-five had some lens changes attributable to age. Another study, The Health and Nutrition Examination Survey (Hanes), conducted by the Department of Health, Education and Welfare and reported in the *Archives of Ophthalmology* in April 1982, found that the age group sixty-five to seventy-five had an average incidence of cataracts of about 30 percent. In other words, of every ten people 65 years or older, about eight will show some aging change in the lens of each eye, while at least three will have diminished vision due to cataracts. I point this out not to make you rush to your nearest ophthalmologist, but to put things in perspective and show that a cataract is just part of the normal aging process.

But if cataracts are a normal part of the aging process, why is there so much variation among individuals? Why does an eighty-year-old get only mild vision problems, while his sixty-nine-year-old brother already has had surgery for advanced cataracts? Why are some babies born with cataracts? Why will a cataract take ten years to grow in one eye and only one year to grow in the other eye of the same person? The answer, at the present state of knowledge, is we just don't know. Many factors have been implicated in causing senile cataracts, from lack of vitamins to prolonged exposure to light, but nothing conclusive has been found. Intensive investigation is being conducted throughout this country, not only in the laboratory but in doctors' offices and hospital clinics. Jules Stein, M.D., the famous musical entrepreneur who founded the Music Corporation of America, established Research to Prevent Blindness, a New York–based philanthropy devoted to research in eye disease and ending blindness, no matter what the cause. A great deal of eye research is supported by this organization as well as by the National Institutes of Health and other private and governmental organizations. That magic pill which will dissolve cataracts and restore 20/20 vision is today in the realm of science fiction, but research is the only means of making it reality.

Dr. Abraham Spector, professor of ophthalmic biochemistry at Columbia University College of Physicians and Surgeons, is one of the leaders in research in human cataracts. He has found evidence of hydrogen peroxide in the aqueous fluid that surrounds and nourishes the lens. This peroxide, identical to the bottled kind available at your local pharmacy, is very likely to be a cause of changes in the human lens that lead to loss of transparency and cataract formation. Why the peroxide forms in the first place is still being investigated.

While the normal aging process accounts, in an as yet unknown way, for the majority of cataracts in the general population, diabetes plays a significant role in cataract formation in the diabetic population. Diabetes, a disorder characterized by elevated blood sugar levels, is present in about 10–15 percent of patients with cataracts, and the most advanced state of knowledge on the true cause of cataracts and possible medical, rather than surgical, treatment lies in the field of diabetes and cataracts. The younger the diabetic and the longer the duration of diabetes, the more likely the chance of developing a cataract. For some reason this is more true of females than males. Poor control of diabetes may play a role in cataract development and this ought to be another incentive for a diabetic patient to be more careful about diet, medication and medical checkups.

The most recent evidence on cataracts and diabetes is based on a study of nearly five thousand people in the area of Framingham, Massachusetts, published in the *American Journal of Ophthalmology* in 1981. The study showed that if you have diabetes and are under age seventy, you have a 30–40 percent greater chance of having a cataract than another seventy-year-old person without diabetes. Past age seventy, the diabetic and nondiabetic have an equal chance of developing a cataract.

Clinical observations of cataracts in juvenile diabetics, people who develop diabetes in adolescence and in their twenties and early thirties, have shown that high and rapidly changing blood sugar, or blood glucose, influences the subsequent development of a cataract. A cataract in a patient with diabetes is often called a *sugar cataract* and looks like an oil droplet. In that terrifying era before Banting and Best discovered insulin as the treatment for diabetes in 1922, it was not uncommon for a juvenile diabetic to develop a sudden, blinding cloudiness of the lens brought on by a blood sugar level wildly out of control. Fortunately, this type of cataract is very rare today.

What finally emerged from studies by Dr. Jin Kinoshita and Dr. Leo T. Chylack is that too much sugar in the blood actually causes cataracts. This was quite a significant discovery, and it advanced our knowledge of cataracts a great deal. Three sugars were studied, two of which were found to have a direct effect on human cataract formation. The first sugar, glucose, is present in ordinary table sugar and the second, galactose, is found in milk and dairy products. These sugars, known as aldose sugars, dissolve into the lens of the diabetic and are converted into substances that cause the lens to swell rapidly with the aqueous fluid surrounding it, like a dry sponge suddenly immersed in water. This bloating of the lens with fluid upsets the delicate balance that keeps it clear, resulting in a dense cataract. The culprit in all this seems to be an innocent-appearing enzyme, aldose reductase, which converts the aldose sugars to a form that can cause cataracts.

Several substances have been developed that can block sugar cataract formation in laboratory animals, and an exhaustive search is underway to block cataract formation in humans with diabetes. Several pharmaceutical companies are trying to develop safe drugs that can block aldose reductase, as this enzyme seems responsible for the formation of sugar cataracts. Perhaps this research can also lead to medical rather than surgical treatment of senile cataracts as well. Let me hasten to add that the majority of people with diabetes will not get any eye problem at all. Good control of your diabetes and regular visits to your ophthalmologist will help ensure that you remain in this majority.

The stimulus for all this work on glucose, diabetes and sugar cataracts actually came from a rare disease called *galactosemia*. This disease affects newborns and occurs in about one out of every eighteen thousand births. It results in severe malnutrition for the baby no matter how much milk he drinks. The reason for the seeming paradox of malnutrition in the face of plenty is the lack of an enzyme which enables the baby to digest galactose, a component of the principal sugar in milk, lactose. Without this enzyme the otherwise healthy baby cannot get proper nourishment, and if the disease is not recognized quickly the baby will die in one or two months.

One of the effects of the undigested galactose is that it is converted by aldose reductase to a substance that accumulates in the lens of the newborn infant in very high amounts and in over 75 percent of cases causes a severe cataract. The ophthalmologist's role is crucial, because the dense, white cataracts are often the first sign of this otherwise fatal disease. Treatment is simple—take the baby off all milk products and substitute soy milk, which lacks the milk sugar galactose. If recognized before four weeks of age, the prognosis is excellent: the cataract will disappear and the baby's health will return.

Although a very small segment of the population is directly affected by the missing galactose sugar enzyme, a much greater segment, children and adults alike, have milder, less serious forms of milk intolerance which may reflect a partial loss of the same enzyme. One of the questions I always ask a young person with cataracts is "How do you like milk?" If the answer is "I like it, but my stomach doesn't," I think of the galactose enzyme. There is no hard evidence of a link between senile cataracts and milk intolerance, but there certainly is evidence for it in juvenile cataracts. The diagnosis is made by several simple blood and urine tests, which should be done on all babies and children with cataracts.

Babies without any milk intolerance at all can still be born with cataracts in one or even both eyes. This occurs in about one out of every three to four hundred births. These congenital cataracts can be small localized opacities in the lens which do not interfere with vision, or can involve total clouding of the entire lens with resulting blindness. We now recognize that if the baby is to regain useful vision in the eye with the cataract, whether it be one or both eyes, surgery must be performed within the first few months of life. You have only to look at the eyes of a two-month-old to appreciate the wonders of microsurgery.

A congenital cataract is usually discovered by the mother, who notices a white pupil in the baby's eye instead of the normally black one. There are many causes of congenital cataracts, the common denominator being something which interferes with the normal development of the lens in the fetus. Medications taken by the mother during pregnancy can adversely affect the developing eye, especially cortisone-type drugs and certain tranquilizers. Premature babies are more apt to have a congenital cataract than a full-term baby. German measles or rubella infection in the mother, especially during the last part of the first three months of pregnancy, can seriously affect the developing eye, causing congenital cataracts in the majority of cases. Fortunately, vaccines can prevent congenital cataracts and deformities from German measles.

Of course, the majority of children pass through infancy without the galactose sugar cataract or the congenital cataract. But they are vulnerable to a more common cataract—the traumatic cataract. This develops from an injury to the eye, either one in which an object penetrates the eye and touches the delicate clear lens, or one which jars the lens enough to damage it. That is why as an ophthalmologist I hate July 4th, with its parades and firecrackers. Out of those thousands of children patriotically and frantically waving their flags, dueling with their brothers and sisters and running back and forth, some will fall. One can hope that at worst the child will scratch his arm, not his eye, but I have seen enough eye injuries to shudder at the thought of another parade. Most eye injuries are not serious, but the exception to the rule does happen all too frequently. I often hear my children muttering "eccentric" under their breath when I caution them about walking about carrying scissors, pencils or anything with an end that even faintly resembles a point. Never, ever, let children play with anything with a pointed end.

Many other causes of cataracts are quite rare and even sometimes bizarre. Glass blowers are prone to cataracts supposedly from constant exposure to intense heat. Electrical workers may develop cataracts from electric shock, and patients who undergo electroconvulsive shock treatments for various psychiatric disorders may develop cataracts. Even other eye diseases such as iritis, an inflammation of the iris or colored part of the eye, can lead to cataracts. Cataracts that result from eye disease are called *secondary cataracts*.

There is some, but so far inconclusive, evidence that malnutrition may play a role in causing cataracts. Malnutrition is often a combination of protein, vitamin and mineral deficiencies, and it is not clear which if any of these factors is responsible should a cataract develop. A fascinating study was performed in 1982 by Dr. Harold Skalka, chairman of the department of ophthalmology at the University of Alabama School of Medicine. He examined 173 older people and found that one-third of them had evidence of riboflavin or vitamin B_2 deficiency. This was nothing new, as previous surveys of nutrition in the older age group of the United States had found the same thing. However, what was interesting was that of the 173 people studied, sixteen of them, or about 10 percent, had an absolutely clear lens in each eye with no trace of a cataract. These sixteen people not only showed no vitamin B_2 deficiency, but had higher levels of vitamin B_2 than even healthy young adults. When these sixteen adults with no evidence of a cataract were matched with fifty-three adults with cataracts, the main difference was in the level of vitamin B_2. This finding was quite significant. It does not mean, however, that everyone over sixty-five should immediately run to his nearest vitamin B_2 supplier, for this is only one small study. But you should ensure that your general dietary habits are optimum, not only for vitamin B_2 but for all sources of nutrition.

Although low levels of calcium can also lead to cataracts, the cause is usually not poor intake of calcium, such as we get in dairy products, but improper working of four tiny glands in the neck, the parathyroid glands. These glands control blood levels of calcium, and malfunction, if untreated, will cause low blood calcium and cataracts, regardless of diet.

Cataracts are fairly common among individuals who must take continuous doses of cortisone or other steroids for such illnesses as arthritis, asthma and gastro-intestinal disorders. Cortisone comes in several different preparations, such as Prednisone, and all forms can cause a specific type of opacification of the back part of the lens just under the capsule. This posterior subcapsular cataract is quite characteristic of cortisone use, and if a patient has been taking cortisone for a long time it may be inevitable. If you are taking cortisone, ask your doctor about alternative medications or lower doses of cortisone. In general the smaller the dose and the shorter the course of cortisone medication, the less chance you have of developing a cataract. Unfortunately there is more and more evidence that even small doses in susceptible people can result in a cataract. You and your doctor must weigh the risks and benefits of cortisone use. If you must be on cortisone, make sure to see your ophthalmologist at least once a year.

Glaucoma sufferers have a dilemma similar to that of cortisone users who risk cataracts as the possible price of controlling another disease. It was known for some time that patients who suffer from glaucoma, an eye disease in which the pressure in the eye is higher than normal, tended to get cataracts more frequently than the general population. Most of the patients with glaucoma took eyedrops called miotics, such as pilocarpine, to lower the eye pressure and thus prevent damage to the eye and preserve sight. However, these same drops which control glaucoma also were found to cause cataracts. Fortunately these cataracts grew extremely slowly, taking up to twenty years to cause symptoms of diminished eyesight, and during that time the pressure in the eye was continuously regulated by the glaucoma drops, like a spigot in a water barrel, constantly letting enough fluid out to avoid a buildup of pressure. With the advent of newer antiglaucoma drops, many patients have been able to switch from the miotic drops to others which do not play any role in cataract formation. If miotic drops are the only ones which will control your glaucoma, then of course you must take them; glaucoma is a serious disease. Should a cataract develop in ten or twenty years, surgery can successfully remove it, as we will soon discuss.

5

How to Choose an Ophthalmologist

Most people have a family medical doctor who is consulted for colds, flu, stomach upsets and more serious illnesses, and a dentist for preventive checkups and dental care. Many women have a gynecologist whom they see regularly, often for nongynecologic problems as well. People ordinarily do not have a neurosurgeon, proctologist or radiologist; these highly specialized doctors are generally required only on referral by a family medical doctor. But, though specialized, the eye doctor is certainly high on the list of doctors most people will see with some regularity throughout their lives. Frequently the eye doctor is an optometrist rather than an ophthalmologist, and since both are "doctors," what is the difference?

An *optometrist* is a doctor of optometry (O.D. instead of the ophthalmologist's M.D.) and is not a physician. He has been through college and four years of optometry school where he learned the basic techniques of the eye examination as well as how to screen for, and diagnose, common eye problems. During his training emphasis was placed on refracting the eye—that is, determining the need for glasses and giving a suitable prescription. He also developed a great deal of expertise in the fitting, formulation and sale of eyeglasses and contact lenses.

Optometrists who are skilled in refractions, contact lenses and dispensing of glasses perform valuable services for their patients. Many patients I see were first told of cataracts or glaucoma by their local optometrist, who then rightly advised the patient to seek the care of an ophthalmologist.

An *ophthalmologist* is first a physician, a medical doctor, just as a neurosurgeon or general practitioner is a physician. The ophthalmologist has been through college, four years of medical school, one year of internship and at least three years of specialized residency training in diseases and surgery of the eye. Some ophthalmologists then go on to subspecialize. This means one or two more years of training in just one type of eye disease. A corneal surgeon who performs corneal transplants or a retinal surgeon who only does surgery for detached retinas are two examples of such subspecialization.

Cataract surgeons are usually general ophthalmologists who develop their skills during their residency training and start a practice after their training is completed. They learn new techniques in courses given throughout the country or by visiting and operating with experts in the field. The major portion of their operating time is spent doing cataract surgery, and while this may seem repetitious and unstimulating, most of the joy in any field of ophthalmic surgery comes from fairly specialized surgery done week after week. The general ophthalmologist will also see patients for eyeglass prescriptions, conjunctivitis, glaucoma and all other eye problems.

Opticians, the third group in the eye-care triumvirate, are trained in taking the eyeglass prescription you get from the doctor, helping you select a suitable frame, and grinding and formulating lenses to make a pair of spectacles. In some states, such as New York, opticians can also fit and dispense contact lenses in the same way as an ophthalmologist or optometrist. They are not trained or licensed to examine the eye, only to make the glasses or contact lenses.

If you suspect a cataract as the source of your eye trouble or if you suspect your problem is something other than can be cured with glasses, you must be under the care of an ophthalmologist. Through medical school and internship he has built up a foundation of how diseases affect the human body, how they progress, how symptoms can be narrowed down to one diagnosis when they initially seem to represent ten or twenty. All this knowledge becomes so ingrained that much of it is subconscious and forms the basis of the most precious skill a physician can possess—judgment. Diagnoses can now be made by computers and surgical techniques can be taught to many technicians, but judgment is a decision-making process that is largely based on subconscious, innate qualities that are difficult to learn. Judgment means being able to tell which patient with a headache needs the aspirin and which needs the neurosurgeon. Judgment means knowing which patient is truly unhappy with his eyesight and needs cataract surgery, and which patient can still function adequately enough to delay surgery and merely needs reassurance and encouragement.

How do you go about finding an ophthalmologist, or any physician for that matter, with diagnostic acumen, surgical skill, impeccable character, good judgment and warm personality? Assuming that you are successful in your search, what happens if you do not like him or her, if there is no "chemistry" between you? It would be wonderful to find in that gifted eye surgeon someone you also like, can talk to and can call at two in the morning without quaking with fear, should there be a problem. Confidence and trust are extremely important in a good relationship between patient and doctor, for without this you may become disenchanted with the doctor in spite of what may be a technically perfect surgical result.

Following is a list of ways to find an ophthalmologist. We will examine each method in detail, as they all have drawbacks.

1. Ask your family doctor.
2. Ask the chief resident of ophthalmology at a major hospital.
3. Ask a friend or relative.
4. Consult the phone book.
5. Call the local medical society.

Referral from Family Doctor

A referral from your family doctor is one of the best means available for choosing an ophthalmologist, but it is not foolproof. Let's say you are seventy years old and have been seeing your medical doctor for five or ten years. You may have initially consulted him for a specific problem such as high blood pressure, flu, or may have needed only a checkup. Over the years you've consulted him for various problems and have always been quite pleased with his treatment and judgment and have developed confidence and trust in him, not only as a physician but as a friend. What better way to locate his ophthalmologic counterpart than to ask him? He will naturally want you to have the best care and would most likely feel personally responsible for his choice of an eye doctor. He should recommend the person he thinks is best qualified to remove your cataract. But will he? Will he truly know the best qualified eye doctor? Will he recommend the ophthalmologist he would use for his own family should cataract surgery be needed? The answer is sometimes yes, sometimes no.

Doctors do not belong to any exclusive medical club where everyone knows the intimate details about everyone else and all band together to exchange vows of secrecy. I would hardly know any better than you the best surgeon in my area to fix a broken hip or do open-heart surgery. I would have to get recommendations from my colleagues and then decide. In the end I would probably have an easier, quicker and more fruitful search than you, but it would still require a search and a decision. This decision would have to take into account one great pitfall: Doctors have friends who are doctors and quite naturally want to help their friends. This is a laudatory trait out of the office, but has no place in the office. If your family doctor is to live up to his reputation, he must put aside friendship and loyalty and refer you to someone he feels is the most competent, friend or not.

If your medical doctor has had your trust and faith over the years, the specialists he uses will merit this same relationship. Since you are probably not the first patient he's had to refer to an ophthalmologist for cataract surgery, he will have formed an opinion over the years about which ophthalmologists his patients seem to do best with and he will have developed confidence in their ability. He should be able to match your personality against the ophthalmologist to whom you will be referred. Most likely he will refer you to someone on the staff of the same hospital as he, so that should the need arise, he will be available to see you in the hospital. You might ask your family doctor if he's had many patients who have used this ophthalmologist for cataract surgery and perhaps speak to one or two of them about their experience. This is much more sensible than asking your ophthalmologist for the names of several people on whom he's operated as his will naturally be a biased selection.

Referral from Chief Resident

The second means of finding an ophthalmologist to take care of your cataracts is probably the best, but it is also the most difficult. Call the eye clinic at a nearby large medical center, preferably a teaching hospital, and request to speak to the chief resident in ophthalmology. You will usually be put through to an ophthalmology resident who is almost finished with his training and who should be able to give an objective recommendation for two or three ophthalmologists he feels are especially skilled in cataract surgery. More than likely he will have operated with these ophthalmologists, assisting them and in turn having them assist him. He should have formed an opinion about their capabilities and be in a good position to provide several names. It would help in getting a more accurate recommendation if you had some idea whether or not you wanted an implant, as one ophthalmologist may be better for cataract surgery with an implant, while another may be better for the more standard cataract surgery. We will discuss implants and other aspects of cataract surgery in Chapter 7.

Lay Recommendation

A third way to find an ophthalmologist is through a recommendation from a friend, relative or neighbor. This can result in a blessing or a calamity, and the odds may be fifty-fifty. The key is the person from whom you are getting the recommendation. Is it someone discriminating and reliable? Was that great internist your cousin recommended the type of doctor you would want in an ophthalmologist? Does your cousin tell you the good and the bad, or is he the type who automatically knows only "the best"—the best Italian restaurant, the best accountant, the best ophthalmologist. Even with the best of intentions, a visit to an eye doctor enthusiastically recommended by a friend or relative may leave you unimpressed. There are several reasons for this: Your son or daughter may have seen an eye doctor for reasons other than a cataract, such as contact lenses or glaucoma, and the doctor may be better for those problems than for cataracts and cataract surgery. Perhaps the doctor does not use the newer methods of cataract surgery or does not use implants. He may not be the right surgeon for you, then. It is therefore a good idea to ask your referral source how he or she got the doctor's name.

There may be two or three other people who have used him and can attest to his skill.

Phone Book

Finding an ophthalmologist by flipping through the Physicians section of the phone book and selecting the one whose location is the most convenient is a poor method of selecting someone to examine your eyes and perhaps operate on them. It is purely a matter of luck if you do fall into the hands of someone you like and can trust to advise you on surgery and remove your cataracts. The Yellow Pages is a terrific way of finding a neighborhood pharmacy or liquor store, but is not recommended in locating a physician. The size of the advertisement has no bearing on the competence of the doctor.

A listing of physicians and surgeons grouped by specialty is, however, a great help when you are in a strange city and need an ophthalmologist, and that, I think, is the main advantage of such a listing. It is at least an excellent starting point in locating a physician when other avenues are unavailable.

If you do find yourself in the situation, needing to locate an ophthalmologist through the phone book, you should ask several questions on the phone. No staff member in an office should hesitate to supply this information.

Is the doctor board certified? While this does not

necessarily indicate the level of surgical skill of an eye doctor, it is some measure of the level of knowledge, since board certification requires passing a series of oral and written examinations after residency training is completed. Board certification should be a minimum standard of excellence.

From what medical school did the doctor graduate? Although I know many excellent physicians who are graduates of a foreign medical school, other things being equal, it is better to see a graduate of an American medical school, since the clinical training is often superior.

With what hospital is the doctor affiliated? Most large cities have teaching hospitals where medical students, interns and residents learn and work and do research as well as teach. Physicians exposed to this educational milieu are often more stimulated than their counterparts in nonteaching hospitals to keep up with advances in their fields. If you are not familiar with the hospital affiliation of the ophthalmologist, ask if it is a teaching hospital and whether or not there is a residency program in ophthalmology. The academic atmosphere of the hospital, clinical skills of the physicians and general patient care tend to be above average at a teaching hospital.

A move to a strange city may be ophthalmologically softened by asking your present eye doctor to recommend a doctor well versed in cataracts and cataract surgery. He may know someone to whom he can refer you, as names have a way of becoming familiar even

3,000 miles away. If he does not know someone in the vicinity of your proposed move, he can consult the *Red Book of Ophthalmology,* a book listing every ophthalmologist throughout the country, grouped by state and city. It gives a brief biography of the physician, including medical school, board certification and subspecialty, if any. This is quite a bit better than taking potluck with the Yellow Pages.

Referral from Local Medical Society

Checking with your local medical society is often touted by well-meaning consumer groups as a good, objective means of getting several recommendations for a doctor. However, an ophthalmologist need only join the society and pay the dues to get listed in the referral service for any specialty he feels like, be it cataract surgery, retinal surgery or glaucoma surgery. No attempt is made by the medical society to verify the qualifications of the ophthalmologist, nor is any follow-up conducted with patients who have been referred to him. Your call to the local medical society will result in the names of several ophthalmologists who feel qualified in the area of concern to the patient and who practice in the patient's vicinity. Not only is this information often inaccurate, it can also give you a false sense of security. A busy, successful, over-worked ophthalmologist may not encourage the few extra referrals from the medical society and may not be listed in their service at all. Any reputable medical society certainly ought to weed out from its ranks of referrals any ophthalmologist found grossly unqualified or unethical, but the patient would have no way of knowing anything further about the ophthalmologist.

There are several simple ways of rectifying the system of referrals from the medical society. The society should run a check on the physicians who want to be on the referral service by consulting with the chairman of the department in which the ophthalmologist trained. His qualifications can be checked against his application and the referral service can then have some confidence in his capabilities. Follow-up cards should also be sent to patients who are referred through the medical society for help in future referrals. Until more quality assurance is built into the system, it is foolhardy to rely on the medical society for locating an ophthalmologist who performs cataract surgery.

Other Selection Methods

Here are two ideal situations for choosing an ophthalmologist to operate on your cataracts.

You've been very happy with your ophthalmologist who has followed the progress of your cataracts over several years. He performs cataract surgery, does implants and has broached the subject of surgery to you, which came as no shock, since you know your vision has been deteriorating and you anticipated needing surgery. This is usually the ideal situation—look no further and stay with your ophthalmologist.

You have a terrific medical doctor who's been taking care of you for several years or longer and says, "Dr. X is an excellent, conscientious ophthalmologist who has successfully operated on many of my patients and I recommend him highly." Go to Dr. X.

If neither situation applies to you, try to get a name or two from friends, relatives and doctors you've seen for other reasons. Then speak to the chief ophthalmology resident at the nearest teaching hospital and ask whom he would recommend from the list, or perhaps get an additional name or two from him. If you live in a large metropolitan area and have several good recommendations, you may even be able to choose your ophthalmologist based on his hospital affiliation or location.

Selecting an ophthalmologist to remove your cataracts should be done carefully, as you must have explicit faith in his judgment and skill. The vast majority of ophthalmologists throughout the country are extremely well trained in this operation and will do an excellent job. You may often hear of the advisability of obtaining a second opinion, either to help resolve a doubtful diagnosis or treatment plan or to confirm what was said by your own doctor. A second opinion may be appropriate if you are not comfortable with your present ophthalmologist, but the second opinion is really your own. After reading this book you will be able to fully understand cataracts and their surgery and will be able to talk to your ophthalmologist more confidently, judging whether his approach and his recommendation agree with your own. You can make as intelligent and informed a judgment as possible about the person who will operate upon your eye. Then and only then can you give a second opinion and confidently select a cataract surgeon.

6

The Eye Examination

Have you ever wondered about all those instruments and gadgets your eye doctor uses? During your eye examination you may be bombarded with bright lights, dim lights, white lights, red lights, green lights, blue lights, eyedrops, lenses on the eye and lenses in front of the eye. Although I try to explain each step of my examination to my patients, I know that it is almost impossible to come away from the eye examination knowing just what your ophthalmologist did to arrive at the decision to operate on your cataract. In order to share in the decision to have surgery, you must understand what is done in the eye examination. This chapter will explain the purpose, scope and procedures of the eye examination. Once you understand that, you will be a better patient. You will be better able to explain to your ophthalmologist what is bothering you and therefore, more importantly, he will be able to help you more effectively and efficiently.

The eye examination consists of five main parts:

1. History
2. Visual acuity and refraction
3. External examination
4. Slit-lamp examination
5. Retina examination

History

Introductions and social amenities concluded, you are in the examining chair. Your eye doctor asks, "What is the trouble?" Your answer will probably be something like, "My vision is getting worse. I have more and more trouble reading and even need a magnifying glass for small print." Or, "I can't recognize bus signs or people in the street." "I can't watch TV." "I can't do my normal work anymore."

Whatever your actual answer, the basic problem that prompted your examination is vision. It is not pain, tearing, discharge or itching, which are common eye symptoms unrelated to cataracts. It is vision. A most important part of the history comes next. "Was this a gradual loss of vision or was it sudden?" Cataracts usually grow slowly, and the accompanying visual loss is likewise slowly progressive. Sudden visual loss should alert the ophthalmologist to causes other than cataracts, such as a hemorrhage in the retina or a detached retina. Hardening of the arteries or arteriosclerosis can result in insufficient blood flow to the optic nerve causing sudden loss of vision. Although sudden loss of vision in one eye speaks against a cataract, the loss of vision may indeed come from that, especially if the cataract is in your nondominant eye. You may be surprisingly unaware of this for years. When you suddenly notice it, you may be in a state of panic and will hurriedly call your eye doctor. The visual loss was gradual, but your awareness was sudden.

Your ophthalmologist will also ask you about pain. A cataract is almost always painless. The presence of pain may mean an inflammation of the eye called uveitis, or an increase of pressure in the eye, glaucoma. Loss of vision accompanied by pain is unlikely to be due to cataracts but can be serious, and you should contact your ophthalmologist immediately.

You will also be asked about your general health, since it can affect your eyes. Diabetes or high blood pressure can alter vision by adversely affecting the retina. It is important to differentiate between cataracts and retina trouble as a cause for poor eyesight. Removing a cataract from an eye with a retina seriously weakened by diabetes may not significantly improve vision.

Visual Acuity and Refraction

After the history is taken, your eye doctor will have you read the eye chart to determine the level of acuity, or sight, in each eye. Each eye is assigned the level of vision corresponding to the lowest line of the eye chart or the smallest letters that can be read by that eye, such as 20/40, 20/70 or 20/200. If one of your eyes can only see the biggest figure on the chart, such as the "big E," the vision for that eye is listed as 20/400. If your other eye sees 20/20, you, as a whole, will see 20/20, but your "bad eye" will still see only 20/400. If one eye cannot even see 20/400, but can count how many fingers your eye doctor holds up, the vision is called count fingers. If the separated fingers cannot even be discerned but the hand can be vaguely seen to move, the vision is known as hand motion. The next worse vision is light perception, or LP, when only the presence or absence of light can be appreciated. The worst vision is NLP, or no light perception, when even the strongest light possible is the same as total darkness. To an ophthalmologist, NLP is the equivalent of blindness. An increasingly dense cataract will naturally give increasingly poor vision, but no cataract can be so severe as to block out light completely.

After your vision is checked, the ophthalmologist will then perform a refraction—trying different lenses to see which combination will give the best corrected vision in each eye. As you look at certain letters on the eye chart, the eye doctor will try different lenses in front of each eye, and you will be asked to make a choice, "Which is better, lens #1, or lens #2?" This often drives patients frantic, since it seems equivalent to a test in grade school. But unlike grade school there is no right or wrong answer. Just pick whichever lens makes the letters look clearer and sharper. The refraction may be performed with a trial frame, a heavy metal frame with slots for lenses, or with a device called a phoroptor. The phoroptor resembles a giant butterfly and contains hundreds of lenses that can be flipped in front of each eye at the turn of a dial. It is usually suspended from a stand or attached to the wall and is moved in front of your eyes at the start of the refraction. Many ophthalmologists have computerized instruments that can do the refraction automatically in a few seconds. This automated refraction will usually be delegated to a technician or assistant, but in the end your eye doctor will still badger you with "Which is better, one or two?" After the best vision for distance is determined, other lenses will be placed over your distance prescription to achieve the best vision for reading. There may be a big discrepancy between your far and near acuity, as cataracts may behave differently at these distances. The level of your vision is one of the best indications of the health of your eye and the severity of your cataract, and is as basic to your eye health as your blood pressure is to your general health.

External Examination

The third part of the eye examination, the external examination, is done with a small flashlight called a penlight. The doctor will look at your eyelids and pupils, and check the eye muscles and eye position. The lids are often prone to a chronic inflammation called blepharitis, usually associated with seborrhea (oiliness of the skin) and dandruff of the scalp and eyelashes. If blepharitis is present during cataract surgery, there will be an increased chance of infection. Treatment usually consists of cleaning the lids with a cotton swab and water followed by antibiotic ointment.

To check the pupils the doctor will shine the penlight into each eye, alternating the light from one eye to the other. Each pupil should equally and briskly constrict to light. An abnormal pupil may indicate another problem with the eye besides a cataract. A cataract, no matter how dense, will not affect the working of the pupils.

Next, the doctor will examine the soundness of the eye muscles, of which each eye has six. He will ask you to follow an object up, down, left and right. The eyes should work as a pair and not be crossed or drifting apart. A cataract in one eye, present for years and years, depriving that eye of good vision, may cause the eye to drift outward, that is, away from your nose. It is important to know if this has happened, because when the cataract is removed from the drifting eye and vision is restored, double vision will result because the two eyes will not be working together. This can be as annoying as was the original cataract, but fortunately the double vision will usually clear up spontaneously as the eyes start working together.

Slit-Lamp Examination

The slit-lamp examination is the fourth step of the eye examination and during this part your ophthalmologist will be able to examine your cataract to determine how "ripe" or mature it is. Another name for the slit lamp is a biomicroscope, a very apt description because it does give a magnified, microscopic view of the front parts of the eye—cornea, iris and lens—collectively called the anterior segment of the eye. The slit lamp is wheeled into place in front of you and you rest your chin on the chin rest and your forehead against a head rest. Your doctor will look through two eye pieces that look like binoculars, and focus a vertical slit beam of light onto your cataract. With the room lights off and the room quiet, you may think you've wandered onto the set of *Star Wars*. By changing the focus and the angle of the slit of light, the doctor can carefully examine all parts of your cataract. In this way, your eye doctor can decide how dense the cataract is and what type of cataract surgery will be best for you.

Attached to the slit lamp is a tonometer, a probe-like device for measuring the pressure inside your eye, the intraocular pressure. An anesthetic drop is instilled in each eye and a piece of paper impregnated with fluorescein, an orange dye, is painlessly touched to the inside of each lower lid. Some of the dye dissolves in your tears and coats the cornea. The white beam of light is then changed to a blue light by flipping a lever on the slit-lamp arm and the tonometer probe is slowly moved towards your eye. As he looks through the slit lamp, your ophthalmologist will see a fluorescent pattern as the probe gently touches your cornea. The force needed to make this pattern is equal to the intraocular pressure. The test is quite painless and simple and need not cause any anxiety. The normal intraocular pressure is usually between fourteen and twenty-one; a reading over twenty-one may indicate the presence of glaucoma. Since cataract surgery is safer when the eye pressure is normal or even below normal, it is extremely important for your doctor to make this determination before your operation.

You will also undergo a test called gonioscopy. In this test, the angle the cornea makes with the iris, the anterior chamber angle, is checked with a mirrored lens called a gonioscope. It is through this angle that fluid drains out of the eye, and when this drainage gets blocked the pressure will rise and glaucoma may ensue. It is important that your doctor do this test, for several reasons. The angle should be very wide open, rather than narrow or closed. If the angle is very narrow, dilating drops can further narrow it and block fluid from leaving the eye, causing a rapid rise in intraocular pressure and acute glaucoma. Just prior to cataract surgery the pupil may need to be very dilated through the use of drops, and if this causes a severe rise in intraocular pressure, complications may result during the surgery. Another reason the anterior chamber angle must be checked with the gonioscope is that an anterior chamber implant, which we will examine closely in Chapter 8, will be held in place by fitting snugly into this angle. In some inflammatory conditions of the eye, this angle is obliterated and there would be no place for the implant to lie. All this can be known prior to surgery by examining the eye with a gonioscope.

If your anterior chamber angle has been found to be open it is safe to dilate your pupils. This is usually done with two kinds of eyedrops—Mydriacyl or Cyclogyl, and phenylephrine. These drops work by temporarily paralyzing the muscles in the iris that make the pupil small and by stimulating the muscles that make the pupil big. This way the pupil is maximally enlarged, facilitating a clear view of the back of the eye. This accomplishes three things. It allows further examination of the cataract, it gives your ophthalmologist an idea how much your pupil will dilate for your cataract surgery and it allows him to look at the retina, the fifth part of the eye examination. The drops will take about a half hour to work, so you'll need to return to the waiting room.

Retina Examination

An examination of the retina may be as important as the examination of the cataract. Both will have a major effect on the decision to operate and the prognosis for improving sight. The retina, the membranelike lining of the back of the eye, is viewed through an ophthalmoscope. The usual ophthalmoscope is a hand-held instrument, something like a flashlight with lenses, through which the ophthalmologist focuses on the back of your eye. (Your medical doctor also uses the ophthalmoscope to uncover any effects of high blood pressure and diabetes in your eyes.) The problem with this instrument is that it does not emit a strong enough light to see through a cataract.

Another type of ophthlamoscope, the binocular indirect ophthalmoscope, is indispensable in evaluating a patient for cataract surgery, because it emits an extremely strong light which, except with a very dense cataract, will allow a sufficiently clear view of the retina to predict if it is normal or not. This is extremely important, for if the retina is not nearly normal, removing the cataract may not improve vision enough to warrant an operation. The indirect ophthalmoscope is mounted on a headband, and with the lights out your eye doctor may look more like a coal miner than a physician. By having you look in different directions, he can examine the entire retina. The denser your cataract, the less clear will be his view of the retina, because the cataract will prevent your doctor from looking in to the same extent it prevents you from looking out.

The eye examination—including the history, refraction, external examination, slit-lamp examination and retina examination—is now completed. If surgery is contemplated, several additional tests may be necessary at this time. These tests are the A-scan, keratometry, B-scan and endothelial cell count. They are especially important if you are going to have an implant, a small plastic lens which is inserted into your eye after the cataract is removed and which functions as your own lens did before it became cloudy.

A-scan

The A-scan is a test to measure the length of your eye by sound waves or ultrasound. The normal length of the eye—from the cornea, back through the pupil, through the lens (or cataract), through the vitreous and through the retina—is about 24 millimeters, or approximately 1 inch. Since you cannot measure this with a ruler, the A-scan machine uses sound waves to measure the length of your eye or, more scientifically, the axial length. This measurement is very important and will enable your ophthalmologist to determine if you need an implant and, if so, how strong an implant to use. The shorter your eye, the stronger the implant has to be to bend the light rays to focus on your retina. In nearsightedness, or myopia, the eye is longer than normal, so a weaker implant has to be used. In severe myopia the strength of the implant, as calculated by the A-scan, may be so weak as to make an implant unnecessary. No patient should have an implant without a prior A-scan.

Keratometry

Keratometry, a measurement of the curvature of the cornea, is also used to help calculate the power of the implant. The more curved your cornea, the more nearsighted will be your eye and the weaker need be the implant. The data from the A-scan and keratometer are fed into a small computer which calculates the strength of the implant needed to give you the best vision. We will go into this in greater detail in Chapter 8.

B-scan

The B-scan is an ultrasound test used in patients with a cataract too dense to permit any useful view of the retina with the binocular indirect ophthalmoscope. A frustrating situation for both patient and ophthalmologist is to operate successfully on a very dense cataract, only to discover that hiding behind that cataract is a totally or partially detached retina. The operation can be a success but the patient still will not see with that eye. The B-scan, more effectively than the A-scan, gives a picture of the eye behind the cataract and can alert the doctor before surgery to the presence of a retinal detachment. As you may realize, this is only necessary when the cataract is extremely dense and when there is a suspicion of a detached retina. Your ophthalmologist will know if the B-scan ultrasound test is needed.

Endothelial Cell Count

The endothelial cell count is one of the best ways to determine the health of the cornea and to predict how it will stand up to cataract surgery. The endothelium is a single layer of cells lining the inside of the cornea, which is bathed in the aqueous fluid in the front part of the eye, the anterior chamber. These cells prevent the fluid inside your eye from entering your cornea, causing it to swell and lose clarity. Such swelling can adversely and permanently affect eyesight.

We are all born with a certain number of endothelial cells, and as we get older some of the cells die and are lost. The cornea has a very limited ability to make new cells and repair itself. What makes this very important is that a certain number of endothelial cells are needed to maintain a clear cornea and some of these cells, about 10–15 percent, are normally lost during cataract surgery, especially with an implant. If only 50 percent of these cells are left by the time cataract surgery is needed, and another 15 or even 20 percent is lost during the surgery, we may dip below the minimum level needed for a healthy cornea. The result may be a successful operation but no improvement in vision owing to a cloudy cornea.

There is a way of counting, with a fairly good degree of accuracy, the number of cells present in the endothelium. This is done with an instrument similar to the slit lamp, called an endothelial cell camera. If the cell count is low, and 1000 is about the lower limit of normal, special precautions can be taken during cataract surgery to minimize the risk of endothelial cell loss. An implant should be avoided, as it carries a greater risk of cell loss.

Not everyone about to undergo cataract surgery needs an endothelial cell count. Your doctor will recognize certain signs when he examines you with the slit lamp that will alert him to perform the endothelial cell count.

All additional tests are completed and now comes the big moment. Are you ready for surgery?

7

Surgery

Until about fifteen years ago, the subject of cataract surgery would have needed only about one-third the space devoted to it in this chapter. There was essentially one type of operation, and your doctor's explanation would have sounded something like this:

"I make an incision into the eye, remove the cataract, and use about six or seven stitches to close the incision. It takes about eight to ten weeks for your eye to heal, and then you'll get cataract glasses."

Today the cataract operation has changed so much, and the events surrounding it have become so complex, that no matter how patiently and carefully your ophthalmologist explains cataract surgery, it can nonetheless be difficult to understand it well enough to make an intelligent decision about when to have sur-

73

gery and what type of operation to have. You cannot leave the decision entirely in the hands of your eye doctor, as well-meaning as he is, since this is an elective rather than an emergency operation. Your evaluation of the doctor's advice compared to your own symptoms will greatly influence your decision on surgery. Most of the responsibility for deciding when to have cataract surgery will be your own, that important "second opinion" of the previous chapter. This chapter will try to clear up the mystery surrounding cataract surgery and help you become a more informed patient. You must make a series of decisions based on the advice of your ophthalmologist and on your own feelings, whether they be gut feelings or feelings of a more cerebral nature. The first is the decision to have surgery.

In the majority of cases the decision to remove a cataract is based on symptoms rather than on the appearance of the cataract during the slit-lamp examination. You, rather than the eye doctor, will know when that cataract is ready to come out. The newborn baby "knows" when the nine months are up and gives unmistakable warning signs that it is time to be delivered. The signs are not as definitive when a cataract is ready to be delivered, but they are discernible just the same if you understand what to look for.

You are ready for cataract surgery when you can no longer see well enough to do the things you enjoy, perform your daily activities in a satisfactory manner and function adequately and happily. When you have cataracts and do not elect to have surgery, you have to accept the fact that although you can function adequately, you may not function optimally. This is a trade-off you must make, weighing your symptoms against the need for surgery.

If your diminished vision prevents you from functioning adequately, cataract surgery is necessary. Of course, what is adequate functioning for one person may be incapacitating misery for another. That is why the level of vision and the appearance of your cataract are less reliable signs of the need for surgery than your own state of happiness in the world. How well you drive a car, watch TV or read a newspaper is more important than how well you read an eye chart. Only after balancing the history of poor vision against the appearance of the cataract and the level of eyesight, can an ophthalmologist advise you either that it is time to have cataract surgery or that the symptoms are not bad enough to warrant an operation. In most cases, allowing a cataract to grow will not hurt your eye or make surgery more difficult later. You have plenty of time to reevaluate your life-style and decide how your reduced vision is altering it.

Certain guidelines have been generally accepted by ophthalmologists to aid patients in determining when surgery is necessary, and these pertain to the level of visual acuity in the affected eye. Certainly, surgery would never be done on an eye with a mild cataract that reduces vision only slightly to levels of 20/25 or 20/30. Vision of 20/40 is legal for driving in most states, so a cataract in each eye causing a drop from 20/20 to 20/40 would most likely be something you could put up with without much difficulty. Vision of 20/50 would be more difficult to live with, but most patients are not too hampered at this level. When vision is reduced to levels of 20/70 or 20/100 you cannot drive a car, cannot easily read a newspaper and cannot look across the street without the sense of a haze or blur. This is the level at which we generally start thinking seriously about cataract surgery, and if both eyes are affected, most patients will go ahead and have surgery in one eye.

If vision is reduced to 20/200 or worse, which is legal blindness, your doctor will strongly recommend surgery. Patients I see with this level of vision because of cataracts and who have not had cataract surgery despite good advice, are usually inordinately fearful of the operation or are denying their illness. It is frustrating to see a patient accept near-blindness rather than have a thirty- or forty-five-minute operation, especially when an ophthalmologist sees hundreds of patients who are blind for reasons no operation could correct.

These general guidelines apply to the average patient with the average cataract, but many exceptions occur. If you are a sixty-year-old accountant or secretary, have a cataract in each eye, reducing your vision to 20/50, and cannot do your work, a cataract operation may be necessary even though your level of vision is not particularly incapacitating for household and leisure activities. Some cataracts, particularly those in which the opacities are in the center of the lens, affect near vision much more than distance vision. This would be especially incapacitating for those people for whom reading and close work play an important part in their life.

In rare instances a cataract may get so big and swollen that it blocks the free passage of fluid from the eye, causing a rise of intraocular pressure. This can lead to glaucoma, necessitating emergency cataract removal, not only to improve sight but to prevent blindness from glaucoma. A cataract can also grow to the point where any further growth will make removal more difficult and would risk the success of the operation. In this situation, surgery would be necessary for technical as well as visual reasons. Much more rarely, this type of cataract can rupture in the eye, causing considerable inflammation. As frightening as they sound, these situations are extremely uncommon and are usually present only with a cataract so dense as to have already reduced vision to levels of hand motion or light perception.

You have decided to have cataract surgery. But which method of cataract surgery is best? Should you have the "old-fashioned" method or the new one with space-age electronics, logic control, computerized function and flashing lights? Do you want your cataract frozen, broken up, emulsified or homogenized? These are some of the options, and a correct decision may depend on your understanding of these methods.

There are three main types of cataract surgery: intracapsular, extracapsular and phacoemulsification. In the intracapsular type the entire cataract with its surrounding capsule is removed in one piece. In the extracapsular operation, the front of the capsule is opened, and the nucleus and cortex of the lens are removed separately, while the clear back part of the capsule is purposely left behind. Phacoemulsification is a type of extracapsular cataract operation in which the cataract is liquefied (emulsified) and then sucked out, with the clear posterior capsule again left behind. We will examine all three methods to see which is best for you.

Before undergoing any type of cataract surgery it is important that you have a thorough evaluation by your regular medical doctor. A physical examination with chest X ray, cardiogram and blood count will detect problems such as high blood pressure and diabetes that can affect the surgery.

Intracapsular Cataract Extraction

Intracapsular cataract extraction is the standard form of cataract surgery, in which the entire cataract—the hard nucleus in the center, the surrounding softer cortex, and the peachskin-like capsule enclosing it—are all removed in one piece (*see Figure 4*). The cataract is removed within its capsule (intracapsular). Those ophthalmic surgeons who prefer the mod-

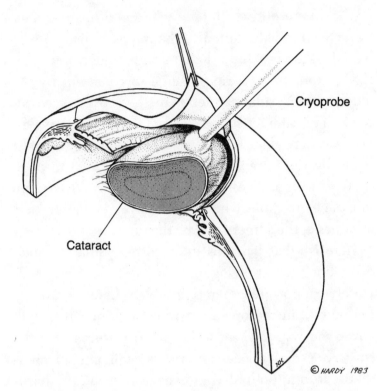

Cryoprobe

Cataract

© HARDY 1983

Figure 4. Intracapsular cataract extraction with iceball at tip of cryoprobe.

ern extracapsular technique sometimes refer to the intracapsular technique as the old-fashioned method, but actually the extracapsular approach dates back to the early 1700s, while surgery by the intracapsular method became widespread only in the early 1900s and perfected in the past thirty to forty years. The intracapsular method, the most popular form of cataract surgery in the world, revolutionized cataract surgery because it allowed the cataract to be removed as a whole before it was totally white and opaque. This gave visual rehabilitation to thousands of people who would otherwise have had to wait and suffer until their cataracts were ripe enough to come out by the older, extracapsular extraction method. If you have already had cataract surgery in one eye and it was performed more than five or ten years ago, it was most likely by the intracapsular method. Let's go through it step by step. Anesthesia will be discussed later on in this chapter, but whether you have general or local anesthesia, the surgery will be the same.

Here is what happens in an intracapsular cataract extraction. You are lying on your back on a firm, moderately comfortable operating table. There are usually two nurses in the operating room, one of whom will cover you with a sheet to keep you warm, and if the surgery is under local anesthesia, will put an anesthetic drop in both of your eyes to prevent any burning when your face and eyelids are washed with a disinfectant solution. A head drape consisting of two or three sterile towels will cover your hair and forehead, and a plastic sheet with an oval cutout will be lowered over your eye and adhered to the skin around your lids. In this way sterility is at a maximum and only your eye will be exposed.

An operating microscope will be wheeled into place over your eye and the surgeon will bring your eye into sharp focus, magnified about four to six times its normal size. Microsurgery is nothing new to ophthalmology, having started in 1947 and come into widespread use by the early 1970s. Prior to the use of the operating microscope, eye surgery was done with the naked eye or with loupes—glasses with an attachment over each eye, giving a small amount of magnification. Most ophthalmologists, myself included, first learned cataract surgery with loupes; it was only at the end of my residency that I learned the fundamentals of microsurgery. The operating microscope was certainly a major advance, as it allowed the surgeon to see minute details he only imagined before.

After the operating microscope is focused, a lid speculum, a small V-shaped metal device, is inserted between your lids to keep your eye open throughout the operation. A suture, or stitch, is passed under a muscle at the top, or twelve o'clock position of your eye, to rotate this part of the eye down into the center of the operating field. The limbus, the area encircling the eye at the junction of the cornea and sclera, is cut at twelve o'clock with a small razor-sharp blade mounted on a handle. Special scissors with curved blades to match the curve of the eye are used to extend this first incision left and right for about 180 degrees. An assistant, either a trained nurse, ophthalmology resident or another fully trained ophthalmologist, will grasp the edge of the cornea with tweezers or forceps and retract it towards six o'clock, giving the surgeon access to the cataract inside the eye. One of my teachers, Dr. Irwin Cohen, observed that the three speeds of cataract surgery are slow, slower and stop. At this point in the surgery his words ring the truest.

Before the early 1960s the most popular method of removing the cataract during intracapsular surgery was to use forceps to grasp the capsule of the cataract and gently and slowly deliver it. A major advance in cataract surgery occurred in 1961, when a Polish ophthalmologist, T. Krwawicz of Lublin, Poland, invented a pencillike device called a *cryoprobe* to freeze to the cataract. When the cryoprobe was removed from the eye, the cataract, still frozen and adhering to the tip of the probe, came with it. This cryoprobe, popularized in the United States by Dr. Charles Kelman, is now used in almost all intracapsular cataract surgery and has replaced the less successful method of removing a cataract with forceps.

As the cataract is removed from the eye, extreme care is taken not to allow any of the inner jellylike vitreous to follow the cataract out. The vitreous occasionally adheres to the cataract and will infrequently extrude from the eye, a situation called vitreous loss. This increases the chance of retinal detachment, glaucoma and inflammation, but modern surgical technique has made vitreous loss much less serious than years ago.

The next step is to close the incision by suturing the cornea back to the sclera. This is done with very fine nylon or silk sutures, more delicate than a strand of human hair and almost invisible without the aid of the operating microscope. Suturing is one of the most critical steps in the cataract operation, as the carefully placed sutures must give perfect alignment of cornea to sclera. If this is not achieved, the wound will heal improperly, resulting in a leakage of fluid from inside the eye and possible infection. If some sutures are too tight and others too loose, the cornea will heal irregularly, resulting in severe astigmatism. Ophthalmic surgeons pay so much attention to detail that countless hours have been spent at ophthalmology meetings discussing the various minute steps of the cataract operation. No other field has been so dominated by one operation as has ophthalmology by cataract surgery.

About seven to ten sutures are generally needed to close the wound. After this is completed many ophthalmologists will give an injection of an antibiotic under the conjunctiva near the lower lid. Although the incidence of serious infections after cataract surgery is very small, about one in one thousand, injecting an antibiotic is generally thought to lower the chance of infection to one in ten thousand.

The operation took only forty minutes and is now over. The cataract was removed whole, within its capsule, intracapsularly, by the use of a cryoprobe. It was painless, whether under general or local anesthetic. An eye patch covered by a plastic shield will be taped over your eye to protect it for the first twenty-four hours. You are on your way back to your room.

Extracapsular Cataract Extraction

Extracapsular surgery began on April 8, 1745, when the great French ophthalmologist Jacques Daviel was performing his usual couching operation on a wig maker called Farian. Couching was then the only method known for removing cataracts and dated back centuries before Christ. In couching, a needle is inserted through the white of the eye and into the lens from the side. The surgeon then uses the needle to push the cataract down out of the line of sight.

The success rate for this operation was around 50 percent, and on this particular occasion Dr. Daviel was unable to push the cataractous lens out of the center of the pupil and was about to face total failure. In what must have been an instant of inspiration and courage, if not near foolishness, he incised the lower portion of the cornea near six o'clock, reached in with a needle behind the cataract and brought the whole cataract out of the eye. This had never been done before, and fortunately the operation was a success. Farian recovered to make many more wigs. By 1750, Daviel was convinced that his method was superior to couching and in 1753 delivered to the Royal Academy of Surgery a historic paper describing his results in 115 cataract operations. By 1756 he had performed 434 operations with only 50 failures, a much better result than in couching. What led up to the extraordinarily refined, beautifully orchestrated extracapsular cataract extraction of today was a series of stepwise improvements in knowledge, instrumentation and surgical technique, so that unless I am mistaken, the extracapsular method of cataract surgery, formerly abandoned in favor of intracapsular surgery, will again be the preferred method of cataract removal. Let's see how it is done.

On the day of surgery, about one to one and a half hours before you're transported to the operating room, your pupil will be dilated to its widest extent by four or five applications of eyedrops, spaced about ten minutes apart. This series of drops is one of the most important parts of the whole operation and actually makes the difference between a smooth operation and a difficult one. The more your cataract is exposed as the iris dilates, the easier will be the surgery. If your pupil is too small, there is a greater likelihood that the extracapsular method will have to be abandoned in favor of the intracapsular one. This is especially true in patients with glaucoma, where antiglaucoma drops may cause the pupil to be permanently small. If you are going to have extracapsular surgery, your ophthalmologist will probably dilate your eye in his office and note beforehand the extent to which your pupil can be dilated, since it is critical to the surgery. Special techniques can be used in patients with a small pupil, but a well-dilated pupil means easier surgery.

In the operating room, everything will be the same as in intracapsular surgery up to the point at which the initial small incision is made into the eye. With extracapsular surgery, your cataract is removed in parts—anterior capsule first, nucleus second, cortex third. In order to gain access to the cataract and intentionally leave behind the posterior or back part of the capsule, the surgeon must first open the front of the capsule. The small incision into the eye, about $\frac{1}{10}$ inch in length, permits the entrance of a thin needle, and a dozen or more little cuts, resembling beer-can openings, are made into the anterior capsule (*see Figure 5a*). This creates a wide opening in the capsule corresponding in size to the dilated pupil. Your doctor will try to cut away as much of the anterior capsule as possible, so that he can remove the inner hard part of the cataract, the nucleus. To do this he has to open the eye a little further, and starting with the original incision, will use those specially curved scissors to create an opening about two-thirds the size of the wound in the intracapsular technique. By applying gentle pressure on the top and bottom of your eye, he will slowly manipulate the nucleus of the cataract so that it slips away from the looser and softer cortex, which remains in the eye (*see Figure 5b*).

Except for fairly advanced cataracts, the cortex is almost invisible without the aid of the operating microscope. If it were not removed it would swell with the aqueous fluid, and by the next morning would turn into a white, fluffy, gelatinlike mass producing a great deal of inflammation. Much of this residual cortex would slowly be reabsorbed over several months and vision would improve, but the results would be far less than optimal.

This slow, almost painful absorption of the rest of the cataract is the reason why extracapsular surgery was abandoned fifty years ago in favor of the more successful intracapsular method. The reason the pendulum has swung the other way now is that the operating microscope gives improved visibility and a more effective way of removing the cortex.

Removal of the cortex is done after the wound is sutured closed, and only five or six stitches will be required as the wound is fairly small. There are two main methods of cortex removal: automated and manual. The automated method, developed by Dr. Charles Kelman, relies on a machine he designed to emulsify the nucleus and to aspirate, or suck out, the remaining cortex. This requires more skill, coordination and dexterity than intracapsular surgery because the surgeon will not only be using both hands to perform the surgery, but both feet as well, one foot to work the foot pedal of the irrigating/aspirating machine and the other foot to work the foot pedal of the operating microscope, constantly adjusting his focus and magnification. He will be doing all this while looking through the eyepieces of the microscope, relying on skillful eye-hand-foot coordination to orchestrate the surgery. To remove the remaining cortex, the tip of a probe is introduced into the eye between two sutures, and by pressing on the foot pedal of the machine, fluid is washed into the eye at the same rate that the cortex

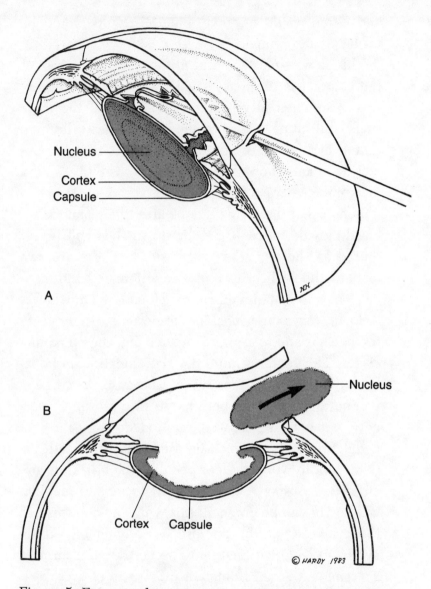

Figure 5. Extracapsular cataract extraction. (a) "Beer-can" openings are made into the front, or anterior, part of the capsule. (b) The nucleus is expressed out of the eye. (c) The cortex is sucked out. (d) The clear, posterior capsule remains.

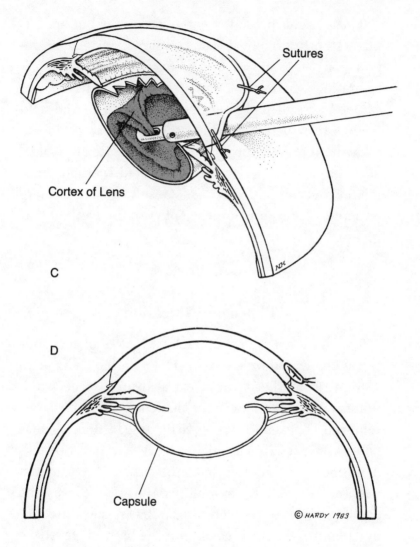

Sutures

Cortex of Lens

C

D

Capsule

© HARDY 1983

is sucked out (*see Figure 5c*). In this way the eye
maintains its shape and volume while the remaining
cortex is removed. The posterior or back part of the
capsule is purposely left behind (*see Figure 5d*).

The manual method is not as dramatic, but accomplishes cortex removal just the same. Instead of relying on the logic-control system of the irrigating/aspirating machine to regulate suction and flow, the surgeon himself sucks out the cortex with a hand-held syringe to which is attached the necessary tubing to allow fluid to flow into the eye as the cortex is sucked out. Although I perfer the automated method, both methods accomplish the same result, and it is more important for your eye surgeon to use the method that gives him the best results.

Phacoemulsification

The third method of cataract extraction, phacoemulsification, was developed by Dr. Charles Kelman in 1967. It is another form of extracapsular surgery and differs mainly in the way the nucleus of the cataract is removed. The same type of irrigating/aspirating machine used for extracapsular surgery is used for phacoemulsification, but this time the probe is a titanium needle activated by a foot pedal which causes the needle to vibrate back and forth 40,000 times per second, emulsifying or breaking up the hard nucleus (*see Figure 6*). Another setting on the foot pedal will activate the suction and the once-hard nucleus, now almost liquefied from ultrasonic vibrations, will disappear into the machine's tubing. What makes this procedure even more attractive is that the entire incision

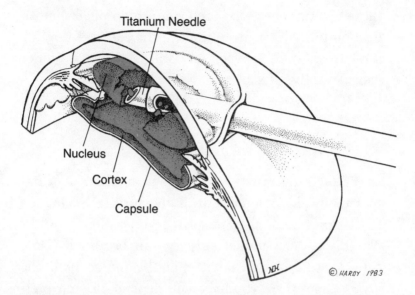

Figure 6. In phacoemulsification, the nucleus of the lens, intentionally positioned in front of the iris, is emulsified by the ultrasonic vibrations of the probe.

into the eye need only be big enough to accommodate the ultrasonic probe, about ¹⁄₁₀ inch. A lot of publicity, favorable and unfavorable, attended the early use of Dr. Kelman's procedure due to a complication rate initially higher than with other methods of cataract extraction. As more and more ophthalmologists gained experience with phacoemulsification, the results steadily improved, although many eye surgeons were still reluctant to attempt it. Today, phacoemulsification is gaining in popularity, and those who use the procedure appreciate the ability to remove an entire cataract through a tiny incision. The extracapsular extraction method appears to be the answer for those eye surgeons who prefer not to do phacoemulsification but who want to remove the cataract through a relatively small incision and still leave the posterior capsule in the eye.

Anesthesia

We have discussed the common methods of cataract removal. As important as the surgical technique is the anesthesia that makes the operation possible. Anesthesia for cataract surgery can be divided into three types—local, local with standby and general. The type of anesthetic you have will depend on your preference and that of your surgeon, your general medical condition and whether your cataract operation will be done on an in-patient or out-patient basis.

LOCAL ANESTHESIA

The local anesthetic is usually given by your eye doctor and not by an anesthesiologist. Prior to surgery you will have received a sedative, and when you arrive in the operating room you will feel somewhat relaxed and drowsy, but awake. This is how you will feel throughout the surgery, the only pain being the mild momentary stinging of the anesthetic injection. Two injections are generally given—the lid block to prevent your eyelids from closing and the retrobulbar block to prevent all pain and movement of your eye.

It would be calamitous if you were suddenly to close or move your eye while undergoing delicate microsurgery, and that is why good anesthesia is so important. The first injection, the lid block, starts in the skin between the temple and the eye and travels up to the eyebrow and down to the cheek. It can also be given near the ear and will have the same effect, numbing the facial nerve which controls the lids. The retrobulbar injection starts in the depression between the cheekbone and lower lid and travels behind (retro) the eye (bulbar). There is absolutely no injection into the eye, as many patients fear, and the needle is thin enough that only a mild stinging sensation is felt. Most of the discomfort of the local injection is the anesthetic solution itself, which burns as it enters the skin. In order to test the effectiveness of the anesthetic injection, your surgeon will ask you to look up, down, left and right and to close your eyes tightly. When no movement of your eye or lids is seen and you have failed all these commands, you are ready for surgery. You will feel absolutely no pain.

LOCAL ANESTHESIA WITH STANDBY

With local anesthesia with standby, the anesthetic injections are exactly as just described, but an anesthesiologist will be at your side to check your blood pressure, pulse, breathing and cardiogram. He will start an intravenous with a mixture of salt water and sugar, not so much to feed you but to be ready should the need arise to give you medication through the tubing. Having an anesthesiologist take care of you will not only benefit your general condition, but also will allow the surgeon to concentrate fully on the surgery. Good anesthesia with a relaxed patient adds significantly to the successful outcome of the surgery.

Once the actual surgery starts, it is not as critical as you might think that you be absolutely still and not talk, but it is certainly helpful to interrupt your own eye surgery as little as possible. Usually you will be relaxed, daydreaming and even sleeping and will wake up at the conclusion of the surgery. The sedation you receive should not induce a deep sleep, since you may awake from such a sleep somewhat disoriented and may move excessively. Your ophthalmologist may prefer that you be undersedated rather than oversedated for your operation. After the operation is over, you will be moved onto a bed and returned to your room. If you are having surgery on an out-patient basis, you have only to change back into your clothes and return home. There will be some discomfort when the anesthetic wears off, usually starting about two hours after the surgery, and two new longer-lasting anesthetics, bupivocaine and editocaine, can even last twelve to twenty-four hours.

With a good local anesthetic and well-performed surgery the total effect on your system is almost like a visit to the dentist. Ambulatory surgery may be helpful for very elderly people, who may feel unsure of themselves in the changed environment of a hospital room.

GENERAL ANESTHESIA

General anesthesia means you are unconscious and completely asleep. An anesthesiologist will start an intravenous through which he will add a sedative, such as Pentothal, to induce sleep. He will then pass an endotracheal tube into your windpipe, through which you will breathe a mixture of anesthetic gases causing you to remain completely asleep and pain free. After you awake you will go to the recovery room for several hours, where a nurse will check your vital signs (blood pressure, pulse and respiration), until most of the anesthetic has worn off. During this time you may be mildly nauseated from the anesthetic and may have a slight sore throat from the endotracheal tube. This quickly passes and by that evening or the next morning you will be back to normal.

The advantage of a general anesthetic, as you may imagine, is that you will not need any injection to locally anesthetize your eye. The disadvantage is that your whole body is affected by the anesthetic and there is a mortality rate of one in ten thousand, especially significant in elderly, frail patients. I much prefer a local anesthetic, reserving a general anesthetic for those few patients who are excessively anxious. You should try to allow your ophthalmologist to use the anesthetic method he thinks is best. It is wise to ask your eye surgeon about this when you agree to have surgery performed. If you disagree with his choice you ought to discuss it with him. It may influence your final decision in allowing him to perform your operation.

Surgical Setting

Where should you have your operation? Five or ten years ago this question would have sounded somewhat ridiculous, as the only place to have cataract surgery was a hospital. You would be admitted on day one, have surgery on day two and go home on anywhere from day three to day seven. In the past few years, several other choices for cataract surgery have become available. Many hospitals have set up programs for ambulatory cataract surgery so that an overnight hospital stay is unnecessary. A survey by the American Hospital Association published in *The Ophthalmologist* in the fall of 1982 found that 70 percent of the nation's hospitals are equipped for out-patient surgery and almost 20 percent of all surgery in those institutions is done on an out-patient basis. The federal government and third-party insurance companies such as Blue Shield and Blue Cross are very much in favor of out-patient cataract surgery because it is easily done under a local anesthetic with little effect on the person's general health or mobility. A federally funded study in 1978 found that as much as a 50 percent savings was possible with ambulatory surgery rather than in-patient hospital surgery. This will certainly be an important consideration for you if you have to pay all or a substantial part of the cost of your operation.

If your cataract operation is to be performed on an out-patient basis you will most likely report to the hospital's ambulatory surgical area on the morning of the surgery and will be escorted to the operating room. Here you will change into a hospital gown and then be helped onto the operating table. Almost all ambulatory cataract surgery is performed with a local anesthetic, and after surgery you will have only to change back into your clothes and return home, using your unoperated eye to see. It sounds ideal, and for many patients it is. But ambulatory surgery is not for everybody. Some patients live alone, are anxious and prefer the security and comfort of the in-patient hospital setting.

On a smaller scale than a hospital, but often more efficient and comfortable for the patient, are freestanding ambulatory surgical centers, sometimes called surgicenters. One of the first of these centers was established in Phoenix, Arizona, in 1969 by Dr. Wallace Reed and Dr. John Ford. There are now about two hundred and fifty surgicenters throughout the country. Designed only for out-patient surgery, they are usually ultramodern with all the comforts of wall-to-wall carpeting, piped in stereophonic music, comfortable lounge areas and a friendly, efficient and courteous staff. Medicare and most Blue Cross plans will cover same-day ambulatory surgery performed in free-standing surgery centers, but to qualify, the operation must not exceed ninety minutes and recovery must not take longer than four hours. This is to ensure that only suitable types of surgery be done in these centers. In order for you to be reimbursed by Medicare, ambulatory surgical centers must be licensed by a state or national accrediting body. At least twenty-five states have such laws. Annual inspection of ambulatory surgical facilities is required by most states, which also require a surgicenter to be within a certain distance of a hospital to deal with any emergencies.

The doctor's office, a newer, more recent setting for ambulatory cataract surgery, is also supported by Medicare and Blue Cross as another option. This "one-stop shopping" does have its advantages, as having your surgery in a familiar setting with familiar staff may make you feel more relaxed and comfortable. The disadvantage is that having the surgery in the same office as you get your glasses checked may make you equate the two procedures. Although this is office surgery, it is the exact same operation, whether you stay in the hospital for one or two nights, have it in the hospital on an ambulatory basis or in a surgicenter. If you do have a strong preference for ambulatory surgery, it may influence your choice of cataract surgeon, since not all ophthalmologists agree on the advantages of this method for cataract surgery. If you have no preference, have the surgery where your doctor is most comfortable.

8

Seeing Again:
Glasses, Contact Lenses
and Implants

The operation is over, a patch and plastic shield are taped over your eye and you are relaxing in your room. If the surgery was ambulatory you may be resting on your sofa or having coffee in the kitchen. An hour or two ago the sight out of your eye was veiled by a cataractous haze, now gone forever. Now that the lens in your eye is gone, and light has a clear pathway into it, what will focus the light into a clear image? The lens accounted for about one-third of the refractive power of the eye, and without it you will fall that much short of receiving a clear image.

An eye without a lens cannot focus and is said to be *aphakic,* from the Greek *a* for "without" and *phakos* for "lentil seed" or anything similarly shaped, such as the human lens. Your cataract operation transformed your eye from phakic (with a lens) to aphakic (without a lens), and if both cataracts are now gone, you are known to ophthalmologists as a bilateral aphake. Cataract surgery in only one eye makes you a monocular aphake.

The correction of aphakia—how the eye sees again after cataract surgery—is achieved in three ways: glasses, contact lenses or intraocular lenses. You should understand all three in order to help choose the one best suited for you. In some ways the method you and your doctor select to correct your impending aphakia is more important than the method you selected to remove the cataract. Once the operation is over you never have to worry about a cataract in that eye again, as cataracts can never grow back. But the way you see with that eye will be with you as long as you live, and an error in judgment may be costly. This chapter will help you understand the three choices and guide you in selecting the best one.

Glasses

Glasses were the only means of correcting aphakia up to about thirty years ago, when contact lenses became available. If your parents or grandparents wore glasses that looked about an inch thick and made their eyes look twice their size, chances are they had had cataract surgery and were wearing aphakic glasses. People did not complain much about glasses then, because they had no other choice and had to wait, almost blind, until both cataracts were ripe enough to be removed. Any vision was better than that, and patients were generally satisfied with glasses. However, as surgery became more sophisticated and cataracts were removed with the intracapsular technique before becoming totally ripe, patients became more and more unhappy with aphakic glasses. Several problems are inherent in all cataract glasses.

1. Magnification. Cataract glasses magnify objects about 25 percent, causing them to appear bigger and nearer than they are. The newly aphakic patient may pour cream onto the table rather than into the coffee cup, seeing it about 2 inches closer than it really is. The whole environment is also magnified, causing you to feel disoriented. Surgery in only one eye may result in an especially disturbing problem because the thick cataract glass over the eye operated on has to be balanced by a thick cataract glass over the other eye. This allows good vision to the operated eye but intentionally blurred vision to the non-operated eye. If the non-operated eye is not blocked out and has a regular eyeglass instead, the brain will get a 25 percent bigger image from the operated eye than the non-operated eye, resulting in disturbing, intractable double vision. Because this is as intolerable as the original cataract, it is inadvisable to combine a cataract glass over the operated eye with a regular glass over the other eye. That is why when glasses were the only available correction for aphakia, a cataract in only one eye, how-

ever advanced, was never removed until the second
eye had a moderately advanced cataract as well so
that it could be blocked by a balancing cataract glass.

Twenty or thirty years ago it was common for a patient to enter the hospital and have both cataracts removed a few days apart. Both cataracts progressed to
a fairly ripe degree of maturity, both were removed
and the patient saw with both eyes again. If a patient
had a mature cataract removed from one eye while
the other eye was normal, he would not want to have
his normal 20/20 eye blocked out by a cataract glass.
In this case he would continue using his good eye and
let the operated eye go uncorrected by glasses. The
operated eye would be a sort of spare tire, ready to be
called into service if and when the normal eye developed a cataract.

2. *Distortion.* If your grandparents or parents were
finally able to adapt to the magnification problem of
cataract glasses, they would still have to contend with
distortion, another annoying feature of aphakic spectacles. Because of the thickness and curve of the cataract glass, there will be not only magnification of objects but unequal magnification, leading to distortion.
This is even more distressing when looking in any
direction other than straight ahead; the further to the
outside you look through a cataract glass, the more
distortion and blurring you get. Aphakic patients corrected by glasses quickly learn to turn the head rather
than the eyes when looking to either side.

3. Limited visual field. Still another annoying change in vision caused by cataract glasses is a marked narrowing of the visual field. With cataract glasses only a small tunnel of vision is clear in front of you, similar to vision through binoculars. Light rays are also bent so much by the strong cataract glass that some rays from objects don't even enter the eye and are bent past it. This blind area, called a *scotoma,* in the visual field of a patient with cataract glasses corresponds to the edge of the cataract glass. Wherever the patient looks, the roving ring scotoma follows him like a shadow, blocking out part of his peripheral vision.

4. Jack-in-the-box phenomenon. Another problem plaguing cataract glass wearers is the jack-in-the-box phenomenon. This is the annoying tendency of objects, hidden by the ring scotoma, to suddenly pop into and out of view as you move your eye away from the center of the glasses.

In the days when glasses were the only means to correct aphakic vision, Dr. Arthur Linksz, a renowned Hungarian ophthalmologist, wisely said "the first complication of cataract surgery is aphakia." Fortunately many patients adapt to the vagaries of cataract glasses quite well, especially with recent improvements in design and optics. Dr. Robert Welsh, inventor of the Welsh four-drop cataract glass, created a thinner, lighter and better-looking aphakic lens, giving less magnification and distortion and a wider visual field. A new cataract glass, introduced in 1980, claims almost no magnification, but although promising, has yet to make a significant improvement in aphakic vision.

Contact Lenses

Contact lenses so revolutionized the correction of vision after cataract surgery that thousands of people have put down their glasses and learned how to place those hard, tiny plastic devices on their cornea. Gone is the 25 percent magnification, the distortion, the scotoma, the jack-in-the-box phenomenon. Vision is back to normal or almost so, and the patient is a lot happier. Patients thwarted by a cataract in only one eye can now have that cataract removed without waiting for a cataract to develop in the second eye. The brain is able to adjust to the 7 percent magnification of the contact lens, so that the non-operated eye does not have to be blocked out as it does with cataract glasses. Patients hampered by a cataract in only one eye, coping with the lack of depth perception and difficulty in coordination, can regain normal vision after surgery by using a contact lens. In spite of these obvious advantages, there are several disadvantages to contact lenses.

1. Handling. Many patients have a great deal of difficulty handling a contact lens. A certain amount of coordination and dexterity are necessary to place a contact lens on the eye, and this is not easy for some older people. Maladies such as arthritis and Parkinson's disease make it almost impossible for some patients to manipulate a contact lens.

2. *Sensitivity.* Although well motivated, some patients cannot adjust to a contact lens and never overcome the initial irritation. The cornea loses some of its sensitivity following cataract extraction; but in spite of this, many patients have difficulty adjusting to a hard contact lens. Newer hard lens material, such as the Boston lens, the Polycon lens, and the silicone lens, as well as better design and improved optics, have made it possible for many more aphakic patients to wear a hard contact lens. Therefore, if you have tried a hard contact lens but couldn't get used to it, perhaps one of the newer materials, which allow more oxygen to get to the cornea, will help you.

The soft contact lens, introduced by Bausch & Lomb in 1971, was supposed to be much more comfortable and allow a greater segment of patients to correct their aphakia without resorting to glasses. The soft lens material, hard and brittle when dry but swollen like a sponge to a soft consistency when wet, is more comfortable and can be worn for a longer period of time, but has several drawbacks.

1. *Lens care.* Maintenance and care are more involved than with hard lenses, because the soft lenses

need to be cleaned and sterilized every day in a small heating unit.

2. *Vision.* Vision is often unacceptably poor when corrected by a soft contact lens, usually because of uncorrected astigmatism. The astigmatism present after cataract surgery is due to an irregularity in the cornea from one suture being tighter than another or one part of the cornea healing differently from another part. A hard contact lens acts like a new, perfectly smooth cornea, while a soft contact lens more or less molds to the cornea, repeating most of the imperfections present. It is not unusual for a patient to wear a soft contact lens to avoid thick cataract glasses, over which he will wear regular glasses to correct his astigmatism. Improved lens design has resulted in better-fitting, more comfortable soft contact lenses as well as some which specifically correct mild to moderate degrees of astigmatism.

3. *Handling.* Switching from a hard to a soft contact lens does not solve the handling problem and in fact a soft contact lens is often more difficult for an elderly patient to maneuver than a hard one.

A major breakthrough in the treatment of aphakia was the introduction in the late 1970s of the extended-wear soft contact lens (EWSCL). This lens, when wet, can become up to 79 percent water as opposed to about 40 percent for a daily wear soft contact lens. The high water content and thinness of the lens allows enough oxygen to travel to the cornea so that continuous wear is possible for months at a time.

It was with some trepidation that I fit my first patient with an extended-wear soft contact lens, and I remember awakening in the middle of the night half expecting a phone call to report a bad result. The next morning I was greeted by a happy patient who also awoke during the night and for the first time since having both cataracts removed had the same good vision in the middle of the night as in the middle of the day.

Every aphakic patient wearing a soft lens, and every practitioner who fits them, owes a debt to companies such as Cooper Laboratories (Permalens), Barnes-Hind (Hydrocurve), American Optical (Softcon), Dow Corning (Silsoft), American Medical Optics (Sauflon) and others for building research laboratories, hiring scientists, conducting clinical trials and spending millions of dollars to develop the extended-wear soft lens. Some problems of lens design, fit and durability still remain, and perfection has yet to be achieved. At the moment the Permalens, the Hydrocurve lens and the Sauflon lens are the three leading brands of soft lenses for extended wear after cataract surgery and have a proven track record in thousands of patients as being comfortable and safe.

Several problems still remain for extended-wear soft lens wearers.

1. Lens loss. One of the most frustrating problems is loss of the lens. If you have ever gone to bed with your lenses in only to awaken with one or both of them on your pillow or cheek, you know how annoying and perplexing this can be. Your eye doctor may try several different lenses—one tighter or one looser, from several different companies—only to have lens loss happen repeatedly. The exact cause of this is not known, although it is probably related to how well your eyelids close during sleep and how moist your cornea is, rather than to the fit of the lens, however perfect it may be.

2. Deposits. One of the worst problems is the buildup on the surface of the lens of material which coats and clouds the lens, causing blurred vision and irritation. We all have protein, mucus and minerals in our tears and on our eye, and these substances can accumulate on the lens and cloud it, the same way changes in the human lens caused by aging cloud it and cause a cataract. Some patients may be able to wear a lens for even a year without any clouding, while others will cloud up a lens in several weeks or even days. The usual cleaning agents for soft lenses are often ineffective in removing these deposits, and replacing the lens with a new one is the only answer. A local condition of the eyelids, called blepharitis, can lead to excessive production of oil and debris, causing soft lens deposits. If you have this problem and have not been successful in wearing a soft contact lens on an extended basis, ask your eye doctor about treatment for the lid problem. More successful contact lens wear should follow.

3. Vision. Extended-wear soft lenses will generally not give vision as sharp as will a daily wear soft lens, but the difference is usually slight and well worth the convenience of leaving the lens in for months at a time. Your eye doctor should have several different brands of soft lenses on hand, because one may be more suitable for you than another. Astigmatism may have to be corrected with regular glasses worn over the lenses. Silsoft, a silicone lens made by Dow Corning, is an extended-wear contact lens for aphakia that corrects moderate amounts of astigmatism. Although initially it may be less comfortable than other extended-wear lenses, it does offer extended wear and better vision in the face of astigmatism.

4. Infection. Although the safety of extended-wear soft lenses has been proven through clinical trials of thousands of patients, on very rare occasions serious eye infections can develop. Many patients who wear contact lenses will develop conjunctivitis, or pinkeye, a mild, superficial infection of the conjunctiva, the membrane covering the white of the eye. This clears quite readily by discontinuing lens wear and using antibiotic eyedrops. Other patients will develop conjunctivitis, not from an infection but from an allergy to thimerosal, a preservative used in most contact lens solutions. Switching to a solution free of this chemical will cure the condition. An eye doctor will be able to ascertain the cause of the conjunctivitis without much trouble. In rare instances, a more serious infection can occur, not of the conjunctiva but of the cornea, and if you try to ignore it and do not see your eye doctor promptly, permanent scarring and clouding of the cornea can result with impairment of vision. This infection is very rare and is usually not serious if the lens is removed and prompt eye care is sought.

Implants

Although contact lenses helped thousands of patients regain good, comfortable vision after cataract surgery, there were still many more patients who could not adapt to a hard lens, could not handle a daily wear lens and were not successful with an extended-wear lens. While many ophthalmologists retained their initial enthusiasm for contact lenses, others took a radically different course in pursuit of the intraocular lens (IOL). This ¼-inch plastic lens, inserted into the eye during cataract surgery, has stirred more controversy than any other subject in ophthalmology and perhaps in all of medicine. The pioneers of intraocular lenses have been reproached by their colleagues, maligned by consumer groups and regulated by the federal government. Unshaken, they persevere in their belief that the best correction for an eye about to lose a cataractous lens is the insertion of a clear intraocular lens. Revolutionary ideas tend to be accepted slowly, and the idea that an intraocular lens can be used to correct aphakia is no exception. Today there is no doubt of the superiority of the intraocular lens over all other aphakic corrections in achieving the quality of vision present in an eye before the cataract developed.

The idea of replacing the human lens with an artificial one appeared in the memoirs of Casanova in 1776. He described a meeting with the Italian oculist Tadini, who showed him tiny crystal lenses that could replace the human lens. Casaamata, an Italian ophthalmologist who lived in Dresden around 1795, was the first one to actually try this. Unfortunately, the glass lens immediately sank to the bottom of the eye and the patient had to wear spectacles.

The modern age of intraocular lens implantation began on November 29, 1949, at the Thomas Hospital in London, where Dr. Harold Ridley implanted an artificial lens into the eye of a forty-five-year-old woman. His idea was inspired by a medical student, who, while watching Dr. Ridley complete a successful cataract extraction, innocently asked whether Dr. Ridley had forgotten to insert a new clear lens. The student had never seen a cataract operation before and thought that was what should be done. It is a tribute to Dr. Ridley that he did not dismiss the idea as nonsense but began to think about the feasibility of an artificial lens inside the eye. Further study led Dr. Ridley to select a plastic, polymethylmethacrylate (PMMA), as the material with which to make the implant. The plastic canopies of British Spitfire airplanes were made of PMMA, and during the early part of the

Battle of Britain in World War II, enemy gunfire downed many British planes. Fragments of the shattered canopy occasionally lodged in the eyes of pilots, and in those cases where it was more prudent to leave the plastic in the eye than risk removing it, the plastic appeared to be well tolerated and did no harm. Since the eyes of these injured pilots were able to tolerate PMMA, Ridley correctly reasoned that it would be an ideal substance for an intraocular lens. His historic operation was a technical success, but owing to an error in the calculation of the strength of the implant, the patient was left extremely nearsighted, her eyesight corrected with thick glasses later on to 20/60. Dr. Ridley attempted a second implant, on August 23, 1950, and the operation led to a similar result. Although there were a few successes, Ridley abandoned his procedure in 1960 because of a high rate of complications. The implant, placed behind the iris into the posterior chamber of the eye, often dislocated and fell to the bottom of the eye or led to severe inflammation and glaucoma.

From 1950 to 1960 most of the great eye surgeons of Europe tried implanting intraocular lenses with only limited success. During this period there were about two dozen different implant designs, each named after the ophthalmologist who designed it, each trying to solve the problems before it. Each one failed, and implant surgery and those who performed it became synonymous with recklessness, irresponsibility and disaster. José Barraquer, one of the most respected eye surgeons of his time, implanted 493 lenses from 1954 to 1960, and eventually had to remove 250 of them because of complications.

Credit for saving implant surgery from oblivion goes to three men—Peter Choyce of England, E. Epstein of South Africa and the recognized father of modern-day implant surgery, Cornelius Binkhorst of the Netherlands. These three men, working independently, were convinced of the potential benefit of implants and were imaginative and innovative enough to design improved implants which worked. The Choyce lens, the Binkhorst lens and the Epstein lens were used throughout Europe from around 1955 to 1965, when they were cautiously accepted by a few eye surgeons in the United States. Over the next fifteen years, as results steadily improved, implant surgery grew in popularity. Today over 75 percent of all cataract operations will involve intraocular lens implantation.

An implant is a small, clear plastic lens inserted into the eye just after the cataract is removed. It replaces the human lens and helps the cornea focus light onto the retina to give a clear image. All implants have two main parts, a haptic and an optic. The optic is the center of the implant, usually about ¼ inch in diameter, and is made of PMMA, the same material as the Spitfire canopy and as that of a hard contact lens. The optic does the work of focusing the image onto the retina while the haptic holds the implant in place in the eye. The resulting magnification from an implant is only 1 percent, a negligible amount. It gives the closest approximation to normal vision possible today. There are about fifteen different implant companies manufacturing over 100 different implants. Despite the variety of implants, they all fall into three general categories based on their location in the eye (*see Figure 7*).

1. Anterior chamber implants. These implants are inserted into the fluid-filled space between the iris and cornea, the anterior chamber. The optic, or center, of the implant lies just in front of the pupil and the haptics of the implant are lodged into the angle between the iris and cornea, fixating the implant so it cannot move.

2. Posterior chamber implants. These implants are placed behind the iris into the posterior chamber, the space between the iris and the vitreous. The haptics lodge into a crevice behind the iris called the ciliary sulcus or may even go into the lens capsule, occupying the exact position of the original cataract.

3. Iris-supported implants. These lenses were quite popular in the late 1970s and gave good results, but are now almost obsolete. Iris-supported lenses are either sewn or clipped to the iris so that they do not move inside the eye. The original iris-supported lens, the Binkhorst lens, worked well, but improvements in the anterior and posterior chamber lenses have led to its demise.

Although an intracapsular cataract extraction with an anterior chamber implant gives excellent results,

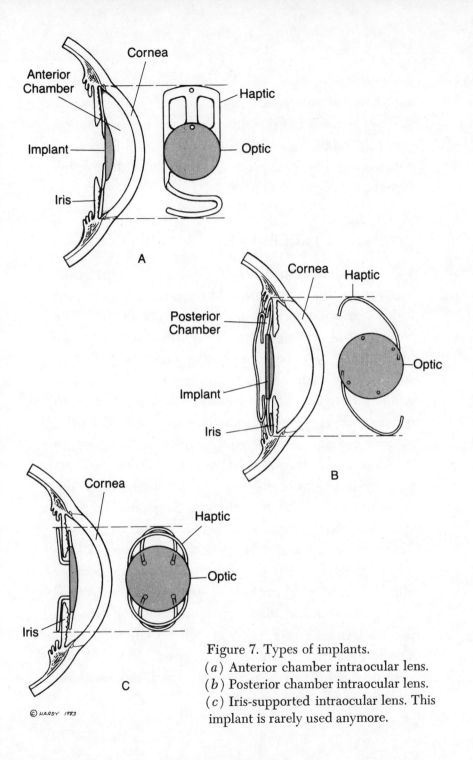

Figure 7. Types of implants.
(a) Anterior chamber intraocular lens.
(b) Posterior chamber intraocular lens.
(c) Iris-supported intraocular lens. This
implant is rarely used anymore.

an increasingly large number of experienced implant surgeons are recognizing the advantages of extracapsular cataract surgery with a posterior chamber implant. It is fast becoming the procedure of choice for cataract surgery, because it closely mimics the eye before the cataract developed.

OPERATING PROCEDURE

This is what happens in a typical implant operation. You are on the operating table about to have a posterior chamber implant inserted into your eye. The front part of the lens capsule has been removed, the nucleus has been expressed out of your eye and after suturing the wound almost completely closed, the surgeon has sucked out the cortex of the cataract. In order to insert the implant, one of the sutures, usually at twelve o'clock, is removed, leaving a ¼-inch space through which the implant will pass. Your eye surgeon will carefully inspect the implant under the microscope to make sure there are no imperfections, since any sharp edges or defects may harm your eye. This intraocular lens will remain in your eye as long as you live, and so it has to be perfect. A meticulous implant surgeon will take your welfare in this regard very seriously, and although manufacturing has improved tremendously, nothing will be left to chance. The implant is grasped with forceps and guided into your eye, helped by a small hook which centers it behind the pupil (*see Figure 8*).

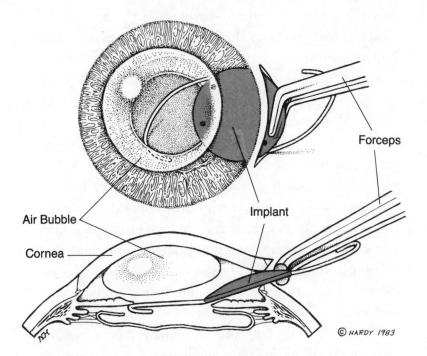

Figure 8. Insertion of a posterior chamber lens implant.

If too much aqueous fluid leaks out of the eye as the implant is going in, the cornea will collapse against the implant and the delicate lining of the cornea, the endothelium, will hit the implant and be damaged. This is the most dreaded complication of implant surgery, as permanent swelling and loss of corneal clarity can result. To prevent this the implant will usually be inserted under an air bubble injected into the anterior chamber through a syringe, much as bubbles are blown through a straw into water. The air will tend to remain in the eye as the implant is inserted and will protect the cornea like an air cushion. If the air, as well as fluid, escapes from the eye, Healon, a clear, thick, jellylike substance can be injected into the anterior chamber to cushion the cornea against touching the implant as it is inserted. Healon, made from the cockscombs of roosters, was originally developed as a shock absorber to be used in the knee joints of racing horses. Its application in ophthalmic surgery has made implantation of an intraocular lens much safer in difficult insertions. If even Healon will not stay in the eye as the implant is inserted and the risk of corneal damage is great, the surgeon will abort the implantation and finish the operation in the usual manner. The patient will be fitted later with an extended-wear contact lens.

The cataract is out, and the implant is in, resting against the clear posterior capsule of your now defunct lens. There is good evidence to show that an intact posterior capsule results in a lower rate of a detached retina as well as less swelling or edema of the retina, problems that affect about 3 to 5 percent of patients after cataract surgery for unknown reasons. An intact posterior capsule in a way "fools" the retina into thinking an operation wasn't even done, and it may lower the rate of retinal complications to less than 1 percent. Unfortunately, within two or three years the clear capsule will cloud over in about 20 percent of patients. Many people ask if a cataract can grow back, and although the answer is an unequivocal no, a cloudy capsule can reduce vision in the same way as can a cataract. We'll learn of a new, simple remedy for a cloudy posterior capsule in the last chapter of this book.

If your ophthalmologist believes in neither implants nor contact lenses, but prefers glasses, I would recommend that you seek another opinion. The quality of vision with contact lenses or implants is far superior to that with glasses. The one exception to this statement is in people who are very nearsighted. The more nearsighted you are before cataract surgery, the more normal will be your eyeglass correction after surgery, since a nearsighted eye has too much refracting power and taking out the lens lessens the refracting power. The A-scan ultrasound will estimate what eyeglass prescription you will need after cataract surgery. If your prescription is a mild one, it does not make sense to have an implant, however small the increased risk. There is still a great deal of controversy among many ophthalmic surgeons whether extracapsular surgery truly does give better results than intracapsular surgery. The most important point for you, the patient, is by what method your own ophthalmologist gets the best results. If an anterior chamber implant and intracapsular surgery is the method he prefers, then you should go ahead with it. The trend towards extracapsular surgery and posterior chamber implants by many ophthalmic surgeons may exert undue peer pressure on others to switch from what they feel confident in to a procedure which may feel uncomfortable and awkward. This can only lead to a poor result. Ophthalmology and medicine in general have been through many phases and the current one will certainly not be the last.

INDICATIONS AND CONTRAINDICATIONS

Implants are not for everybody; your ophthalmologist will tell you if one is advisable for you. The following guidelines, admittedly conservative by today's standards, taken from Dr. Norman Jaffe's *Cataract Surgery and Its Complications* (C. V. Mosby Co., St. Louis, 1976), will help you decide if you are a candidate.

1. Implants should be restricted to older people, generally those over sixty-five. Not enough is known about the effects, if any, of an intraocular lens on the eye over thirty to forty years, a possible life expectancy of a person forty-five or fifty when the operation is performed. More and more patients now have had implants in their eyes for twenty years or more without any harm, but conceivably the plastic in the eye could change over a longer period. The implant material is felt to be so safe, though, that the Bureau of Medical Devices of the FDA is considering removing the sixty-year minimum age requirement for approved intraocular lenses.

Younger people will also have an easier time with contact lenses, and usually if you can wear a contact lens, an implant is not indicated. Unfortunately it is often impossible to know how successfully you will adapt to a contact lens, even an extended-wear one, until one or two months after the surgery, when you actually try a contact lens. If you are not successful, inserting an implant into your eye will require a second operation. This secondary implant carries the same slight risks as a primary implant inserted at the time of cataract surgery, and should be used only as a last resort after repeated attempts at contact lens wear. Patients with a successful secondary implant are among the most grateful and happy of all implant patients, because they have been through the tribulations of wearing a contact lens and now have something with which to compare it. If you have had difficulty with contact lenses I urge you to return to your eye doctor for another try, because improvements are constantly made in lens design and fitting technique. If all else fails, then you should consider a secondary implant.

2. Intraocular lenses should be restricted to one eye only. Until ophthalmic surgeons had more confidence in intraocular lenses this was a fairly rigid rule. It was safer to perform an implant in one eye, and then when cataract surgery was required in the second eye, to fit an extended-wear lens. However, the reverse was often true—a patient was already wearing a contact lens in one eye, and when the second eye required cataract surgery an implant would be inserted. These patients were in a unique position, being able to report their preference for the eye with the implant versus the eye with the contact lens. The impression of most implant surgeons, and admittedly impressions are not scientific conclusions, was that most of these patients preferred the vision and convenience of an intraocular lens. In fact, not infrequently these patients requested a secondary implant in the eye with the contact lens.

If you already have had a successful implant in one eye and need cataract surgery in your other eye, your own ophthalmologist can help you decide on a contact lens or implant for the second eye. With modern, well-performed cataract surgery, most ophthalmic surgeons advise an implant for both eyes, because most complications appear to be due to the surgery itself and not to the presence of the implant. Usually six months will go by before your second implant is performed, to ensure that the first implant is perfect.

3. Several special situations make intraocular lenses preferable to contact lenses. For example, if your occupation or hobby takes you into a dusty environment or underwater, contact lenses may be impractical. I recently performed an implant on a fifty-eight-year-old construction worker who was looking forward to sailing and diving in his retirement. Although we both realized he was fairly young for an implant, it was the most practical approach and worked out quite well.

4. If your first cataract operation was performed without an implant and you are happy with glasses, the second eye should be corrected the same way. In fact, if you have had successful cataract surgery in one eye, cataract surgery in your other eye can generally be deferred quite awhile. Many older people can manage exceedingly well when vision is restored to one eye, and only when their life-style would be significantly improved by good vision in the second eye need another cataract operation be performed.

5. *Implants are usually better for cataract patients with macular degeneration.* Macular degeneration, a disease of the retina common in older patients, causes a loss of central, or straight-ahead, vision. Sufferers of this disease have a great deal of difficulty reading, but can get about fairly well by relying on peripheral vision. Since wearing cataract glasses diminishes peripheral vision, these patients do best with an implant. An important advantage of an implant in these cases is that the implant can be ordered much stronger than required, making patients with macular degeneration nearsighted and thus improving their near, or reading, vision.

6. *Do not have an implant if you have had a poor result related to the implant in one eye or if you have only one eye.* If you have only one eye, the slight risk of an implant is not worth taking.

7. *You should consider not having an implant if there are other serious problems with your eye.* Severe glaucoma, corneal disease or retina trouble from diabetes may be more difficult to treat in the presence of an implant.

Most of these guidelines do not apply in all cases. As more and more experience is gained in implant surgery, many ophthalmologists are lowering the age requirement and performing more implants. An understanding of all the implications of implant surgery plus a thorough and frank discussion with your ophthalmologist should help you arrive at the proper decision.

FDA STUDY

In May 1976 Congress passed the Medical Device Amendment of the Drug, Food and Cosmetics Act, setting up a separate section of the Food and Drug Administration to regulate and control medical devices such as sutures, heart valves, hip and knee joints and intraocular lenses. Prior to this the FDA was concerned mainly with drugs, but because of the plethora of artificial devices, the FDA rightly wanted to assess their safety and effectiveness before we all became bionic. Congress did not suspend the use of intraocular lenses but asked that they be made "reasonably available" on an "investigational basis" to physicians meeting "appropriate qualifications."

It was not until February 9, 1978, that the FDA study of intraocular lenses started. It is probably the largest clinical FDA study ever devised, compiling data on almost a million implants, and will likely extend through 1984 or 1985. The FDA is hoping to amass enough data to decide on the safety and effectiveness of intraocular lenses. Because of this study several FDA requirements have to be met by surgeon and patient alike before an implant can be performed:

1. Each ophthalmologist who wants to implant intraocular lenses must have assisted at implant surgery and developed the necessary skills for this specialized operation. He must register separately with each company whose implants he wants to insert.

2. Because many intraocular lenses are still under investigation, the patient must sign a consent form which explains the risks of intraocular lenses. Most consent forms will scare you if you read them carefully, as you should, but as Dr. James Green, chairman of the department of OB-GYN at St. Barnabas Medical Center in Livingston, New Jersey, said, speaking about another issue, "It is not the art of medicine to scare people to death." More and more implants have been taken off investigational status as enough data has been accumulated to demonstrate their safety, and these are available to any ophthalmologist regardless of training. They will not require a special consent form.

3. After intraocular lens surgery, you should receive an identification card showing what type of implant was inserted, the name of the manufacturer, date of surgery and name of the surgeon. In case you move or need medical care when traveling, you will have a record of your implant. A copy of this card is sent to the manufacturer.

4. Any adverse reactions, however rare they may be, such as infection or severe inflammation, must im-

mediately be reported to the manufacturer, whose records are periodically reviewed by the FDA.

On December 1, 1981, almost four years after this massive study began, the Choyce Mark VIII and IX anterior chamber implants by Coburn Optical Industries became the first intraocular lenses to be taken off investigational status by the FDA. As of May 1, 1983, the following implants have been approved by the United States Food and Drug Administration:

IOLAB
- Shearing Planar Posterior Chamber lenses (models 101, 101B, 101T)
- Shearing Angled Posterior Chamber lenses (models 101K and 105B)

PRECISION COSMET
- Tennant and Kelman Type II Anterior Chamber lenses

COOPERVISION
- J-Loop Planar (model B-13F) Posterior Chamber lens
- J-Loop Angular (model B-1H) Posterior Chamber lens

COBURN
- Choyce Mark VIII Anterior Chamber lens
- Choyce Mark IV Anterior Chamber lens
- Binkhorst Iris Clip lens
- Fyodorov Iris Fixated lens

CILCO

- Shearing Planar Posterior Chamber lens (models PC11 and PB11)
- Shearing Angle Posterior Chamber lens (models PC12 and PB12)
- Simcoe Posterior Chamber lens (models S2 and S2-B)

INTERMEDICS

- J-Loop Posterior Chamber lens (models 019C, K, B, J, F, E)

Implants that are still "investigational" are not necessarily less safe than those off investigational status. It is generally just a matter of time before enough data for each lens is reviewed by the FDA after which the implant is made freely available to all ophthalmologists and their patients. Your ophthalmologist will have up-to-date information on all intraocular lenses.

9

Recovery:
The Postoperative Period

The postoperative period starts as soon as you leave the operating room and lasts until your eyes are completely healed. It can take as little as three or four weeks or as long as twelve weeks. It is an exciting period, as your vision increasingly clears. The morning after surgery your doctor will take off your eye patch and shield. You may see less well than you did before your operation, and you may be upset about this, but it is perfectly normal, even with an implant. After the doctor examines your eye he will undoubtedly assure you that everything is in order. No matter how many times I've removed the patch on that first postoperative day, I never get over the thrill of seeing my patient's eye for the first time after surgery. A brief glimpse with a penlight is usually enough to judge that everything is indeed in order.

Reactions to Surgery

During the postoperative period you will probably experience some of the following reactions to your surgery.

1. Pain. Cataract surgery can lead to as great a variety of symptoms as there are people. Some pain is normal, but what may be annoying pain for one person may be a trifling discomfort for another. Postoperative pain is usually relieved by nonprescription pain medication. Most local anesthetics will wear off an hour or two after surgery and pain will usually be worse then. By the evening of surgery you will be much more comfortable and the mild aching should not prevent a normal night's sleep. Mild pain, as if you had an eyelash in your eye, is also common and usually means you are feeling one of the sutures. This also should clear in a day or so. Severe pain is quite unusual and should be reported to your doctor promptly.

2. Floaters and flashes. For several days, weeks or even months after cataract surgery you may see black spots or other shapes in your line of sight or off to one side. You may even think you see a fly or bug, only to see it disappear on turning your head. A flash of light may appear off to the side like a streak of lightning or the discharge of a flashbulb. These are very common symptoms and stem from changes in the vitreous, the jellylike interior of the eye. After the cataract is removed, the vitreous will tend to shrink away from the back of the eye and move towards the front, taking up some of the space occupied by the cataract. This movement is seen as black spots or lines, and if the vitreous pulls on the retina, to which it is loosely attached, it may discharge some cells just as light does on entering the eye. Hence the flash of light. On very rare occasions the movement of the vitreous away from the retina may pull off a piece of the retina and cause a detached retina. Fluid from inside the eye will flow through the tear, travel behind the retina and peel it off like old wallpaper. About 2 to 3 percent of all patients undergoing cataract surgery develop a detached retina no matter how successful the surgery or how skilled the surgeon. This may happen months or years afterward. Periodic checkups can detect the torn retina before the detachment starts. Such symptoms of a torn retina as floaters and flashes of light will, in the vast majority of cases, indicate merely a movement of the vitreous and not a detached retina. Your eye doctor will be able to differentiate the two by examining your eye.

    3. Tearing and discharge. These are common nonspecific symptoms through which the eye is voicing some protest over being disturbed. The tearing should be quite mild and should require nothing more than a gentle dab with a clean tissue or cotton ball. The discharge, mainly mucus production, will be present mostly in the morning on awakening and should be gently wiped away with a wet gauze or tissue. If tearing and discharge is anything more than mild, contact your ophthalmologist.

4. Light sensitivity. Naturally more light will be entering your eye after the cataract is removed, and you may find it slightly uncomfortable until you adapt to this change. Your own lens also filtered out ultraviolet light, and although sunglasses and some implants will do this to a limited degree, they are not as good as your own natural lens. As the eye becomes less inflamed it will become much less light sensitive. A good pair of sunglasses will eliminate almost all of the discomfort from bright light.

5. Restriction of Activity. Restriction of activity after a well-performed cataract extraction will vary greatly, depending on the judgment of your doctor. Thirty years ago, before the development of sutures, there was nothing with which to close the incision into the eye and the patient had to lie almost immobile for weeks while the incision healed enough to permit any activity—even getting up to eat and going to the bathroom. If activity began too soon, the wound might open and fluid inside the eye would leak out, inviting infection and glaucoma. Modern-day suturing techniques result in a tightly closed wound, and most surgeons permit almost normal activity the day after surgery. This is true whether or not you had a small incision with phacoemulsification, the somewhat larger one with an extracapsular cataract operation or the largest one with an intracapsular cataract operation. I permit my own patients to bend, lift, read, shower and do all of their usual daily activities. At bedtime a plastic or metal shield is taped over the eye to protect it, lest you rub it or lie on it during sleep (*see Figure 9*). This is usually necessary for several weeks, but with phacoemulsification the incision is so small that a shield may only be needed for a few days. Be sure to follow your own doctor's advice.

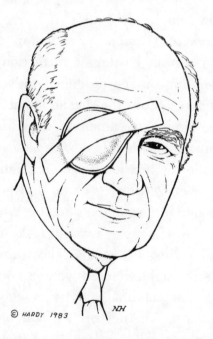

© HARDY 1983 NH

Figure 9. Correct way to wear the shield and tape.

Medication and Office Visits

After cataract surgery your ophthalmologist will prescribe certain eyedrops and medications. These are the most common ones.

1. *Cortisone (steroid).* After any type of cataract operation, there will be a certain amount of inflammation inside the eye. With the aid of magnification from the slit lamp, your ophthalmologist can see tiny white blood cells in the aqueous fluid of your eye. The slit beam of light passing through the fluid will show a smoky appearance, like real smoke in a darkened theater when it drifts into the beam of the movie projector. The more white blood cells in the aqueous fluid the smokier the light will appear. Cortisone and other steroid eyedrops are used to clear up this inflammation which generally lasts from four to six weeks. The word "cortisone" often makes people uneasy, because significant side effects can occur when taken by mouth. In eyedrop form cortisone has virtually no general side effects and is extremely effective not only in aiding healing, but in quickly alleviating any symptoms of discomfort. Steroid drops are prescribed under many different brand names, such as Pred-Forte, Inflamase, Econopred and Decadron.

2. *Antibiotics.* Antibiotic drops are often given for several weeks in the belief that they will lessen the

minuscule chance of infection. Antibiotic drops are actually more effective in preventing infection when given just before surgery rather than after, but it is common to use them in the postoperative period on the theory that "it can't hurt." Many eye surgeons will inject an antibiotic on the inside of the lower lid at the very end of surgery, since this does help lessen the chance of infection. The injection may cause some soreness and swelling in this area, but that will disappear in two or three days as the antibiotic is absorbed. Antibiotic drops commonly prescribed include Garamysin, Chloroptic, Tobrex, Econochlor and Neosporin.

3. *Dilating drops.* Drops that open the pupils, such as Mydriacyl, Cyclogyl and Hyosine, are used before surgery to allow easier access to the cataract, and after surgery to fight inflammation, alleviate discomfort and prevent the iris from adhering to the implant or vitreous. With older implants, such as the iris-plane type, the pupil cannot be fully dilated for fear of dislocating the implant, but since an anterior or posterior chamber implant will not dislocate when the pupil dilates, these drops can be used postoperatively. They not only aid in healing, but also allow the ophthalmologist to get a good look at the retina.

4. *Drops to lower intraocular pressure.* The pressure inside the eye may rise for the first few days or weeks after cataract surgery, and drops such as Timoptic or pills such as Diamox may be needed to lower the pressure. A very high pressure may cause fluid to leak

out of the eye, making you more susceptible to infection. In about 30 percent of people, cortisone drops will cause a temporary rise in intraocular pressure, usually appearing several weeks after surgery. Timoptic or Diamox will usually suffice to lower the pressure until the cortisone drops are stopped and the pressure goes down on its own.

Within a week after the surgery your ophthalmologist will check the progression of healing and improvement in vision. Most of the tests performed then will be identical to those of the examination before surgery, but now you will have the excitement of reading the eye chart with your operated eye. If you are a bit disappointed, do not worry; your vision may still be blurred from inflammation inside the eye, a cloudy cornea and a lot of astigmatism arising from irregular healing of the cornea. This will all subside over the next few weeks and your vision will improve daily. This first postoperative visit is intended more to detect any complication than to determine the best vision in the operated eye.

After you read the eye chart as far down as you can, a brief refraction will be performed to get your best corrected vision. If you did not have an implant, your vision will temporarily be quite blurry until you get glasses or a contact lens. During the refraction you will get some idea of how your vision will improve in your formerly cataractous eye. The sensation should be quite elating. An implant will allow you to see moderately well within a few days of cataract surgery, whereas you would have had to wait several weeks for your eye to heal before getting a contact lens. After the refraction the doctor will examine your eye under the slit lamp, check your intraocular pressure and look at the retina. This will be his first clear view into your eye since you developed the cataract, and he will be able to tell you if your retina is healthy or not. About 10 percent of patients with cataracts also have retina trouble in the form of macular degeneration, an aging change of that part of the retina that gives you clear, sharp vision. With a healthy retina you will have almost no impediment to normal vision, but with macular degeneration the vision will undoubtedly be better than before surgery though some impairment will still be present.

The number of postoperative visits will depend on the progress of healing of your eye and the philosophy of your doctor. Most doctors feel comfortable with three or four checkups over the next six weeks, while others may want to see you almost every week to ensure early detection of any complications. By your sixth postoperative week your eye should generally be free of redness and should feel comfortable. Some additional healing and change may occur up to six months later, but in general, six to eight postoperative weeks is the time for your final refraction and glasses. This point is reached when from one visit to the next there has not been much change in your refraction, indicating that the healing process is over and your vision is stable.

If you have an implant, chances are you will still need glasses to wear over the implant to correct any remaining near- or far-sightedness or any astigmatism. They will fine tune your distance vision to its maximum. Reading glasses will also be necessary, because an implant cannot change shape to focus from distance to near.

If a lot of astigmatism is present, due to a tight suture or unequal healing of the incision, your doctor will probably want to cut that suture and allow the cornea to return to a more normal, rounded shape. This takes a few seconds, is painless and is done at the slit lamp with an anesthetic drop. The less astigmatism you have after cataract surgery, the clearer and more comfortable will be your vision. This is especially important with soft contact lenses, since they correct only small amounts of astigmatism and glasses may be needed to correct the rest.

Should it be necessary to have one or two sutures cut, you will have to wait another two to three weeks before getting glasses to allow your cornea to change to a more normal shape. Be patient, as the one who ultimately benefits is you. If you are to wear spectacles, your final refraction will be written down and you will go to your optometrist or optician for a pair of glasses, either bifocals or separate glasses for near and far vision. If you are to wear a contact lens, you are ready for a fitting.

Contact Lens Fitting

Given the choice, most people over age sixty or seventy choose an extended-wear soft contact lens rather than a daily wear hard or soft lens because of the convenience of leaving the lens in for months at a time. The clearest vision is achieved by a hard lens, and next clearest by a daily wear soft lens, but these require daily insertion and removal, a skill that tends to get more difficult with age. The fitting procedure for the three types of contact lenses is fairly similar and starts with a measurement of the curve of the cornea. This is done with the keratometer, the same instrument as described in Chapter 6 for calculating the power of an implant.

Contact lenses can be fit and dispensed by ophthalmologists or optometrists and in some states, such as New York, by opticians. Some ophthalmologists defer your contact lens fitting to an optometrist or optician who specializes in contact lenses. Others feel that the fitting should be performed in the ophthalmologist's office, because this is really an extension of the surgery. Your cataract operation may have taken only a half hour, your postoperative course may have lasted eight weeks, but your contact lens care will be with you forever. A good relationship with the person who fits you is important, since you may be a frequent visitor to his office, especially in the beginning of contact lens wear. A well-fitting contact lens is as important to the success of your surgery as good surgical technique.

After the curvature of your cornea is determined, a sample contact lens that matches this curve is placed on your cornea. The power, or strength, of the lens will be based on, but not identical to, your eyeglass prescription, so you will see fairly well with only the fitting lens. The clearest vision will come when your eye doctor performs a refraction over the contact lens, and with some jiggling and juggling of the lens will get you the sharpest vision your eye will allow.

The fit of the lens, also crucial to success, will be checked next, with the aid of magnification from the slit lamp. A well-fitting contact lens should move a little when you blink but should not slip or slide excessively when you look up. During the initial fitting, the mild discomfort from having something foreign in your eye is perfectly normal, and will almost disappear within an hour or two. Based on the fit of the trial lens, your eye doctor will order your own contact lens in the correct curve, size and prescription. A great deal of judgment goes into his selection, not only of the fit but of the brand and style of lens. The fitting of your contact lens should be one of the high points of your recovery. You put up with the cataract, had the surgery, waited a few weeks to let your eye heal and now you can finally see well. Although the contact lens will magnify objects 7 percent, you will probably not notice this and the vision will feel natural and comfortable. You may have to wear ordinary glasses

over the contact lens to correct any remaining astigmatism, and reading glasses or bifocals will be needed
for close work. This is true with contact lenses and
with implants.

If you received an extended-wear soft lens, you will
sleep with it and should have no more than minor discomfort or awareness that night. Many doctors will
want to see you the following day, because some problems show up within twenty-four hours. If the lens fits
too tightly, the eye may be irritated and it is best to
switch immediately to a looser lens. A lack of oxygen
caused by a lens that is too tight creates swelling
(edema) and irritation of the cornea, and your eye
doctor will look for any early signs of this during follow-up visits.

After three or four months of lens wear, your doctor
may see you again to see if the lens needs cleaning.
Under the slit lamp, he can inspect the surface of the
lens on your eye for protein, mucus or mineral deposits, and if the lens is clean you may be able to wear it
for even a year or more without taking it out. Drops to
keep the lens moist will help keep it comfortable and
clean and will keep your vision clear.

The main complication, albeit a rare one, of extended-wear soft lenses is infection of the cornea.
It is not that uncommon to develop mild conjunctivitis, or pinkeye, a generally harmless infection of the
conjunctiva marked by redness and discharge from
the eye. To treat this your doctor will most likely remove the lens and start you on antibiotic drops for a

few days. A new lens will be ordered and you should be back to normal in a week. A much more serious condition is an infection of the cornea. This may start as a mild "foreign body" feeling and in a day or two progress to pain, blurred vision and light sensitivity. Such an infection may permanently scar your cornea, reducing your vision considerably. It is very rare and need not cause any lasting damage if promptly treated. Patients get into trouble by ignoring symptoms, hoping it's just pollution, makeup or allergy, and waiting until the infection has gotten a lot worse before seeing a doctor.

Once you are wearing contact lenses or glasses or both, and your doctor has told you he doesn't have to see you for four, five or even six months, your postoperative period is over. Barring any eye problems such as retina trouble or glaucoma, you should now be able to read and drive a lot easier, watch television and do all the other things you enjoy. If retina trouble such as macular degeneration is present, this will limit the improvement in your vision, but some improvement should be present. Significant retina trouble may require you to use low-vision aids such as magnifying glasses, high-intensity lighting and telescopic devices to supplement the improvement from your cataract operation.

We have now surveyed the present state of our knowledge and skills in dealing with cataracts and the optical correction of the eye without its own natural lens. Ten or twenty years from now our current techniques may all seem primitive, but by keeping abreast of advances in the field of cataracts and implants, your ophthalmologist will be in a position to give you the best care possible. Let's see what the future may hold.

10

What the Future Holds

Having given an account of our present knowledge of cataracts and cataract surgery, I want to look to the future, for the knowledge of cataracts and cataract surgery will surely change. Let's see what's on the horizon.

Nonsurgical Treatment of Cataracts

The only treatment for a cataract is to remove it surgically. Although that will continue to be true for some time, a great deal of research is underway to discover an alternative—a medical treatment for cataracts such as a pill taken like a daily vitamin. This research formally began in 1976, when twenty-three research laboratories throughout the United States agreed to pool their knowledge and resources into the Cooperative Cataract Research Group (CCRG). In 1980 this research was consolidated into seven centers with funding from the National Institutes of Health.

Before studying possible cures for cataracts, scientists have to learn how cataracts form, how they block light and how fast they grow. Once this is known, anticataract drugs can be tested and the results evaluated. Research led by Dr. Clifford Harding, professor and director of research in ophthalmology at Kresge Institute in Detroit, and Dr. Leo T. Chylack, Jr., of Harvard University, has resulted in the examination and classification of over five thousand human cataracts. Human clinical drug trials are scheduled to begin in the United States in late 1983, using several anticataract agents not yet generally available. Included among the experimental drugs will be at least one that might prevent cataract formation in diabetic patients, who are at higher risk of developing cataracts than the general population. It will be at least five years before even preliminary results are available, so don't cancel your cataract operation just yet.

Another area of study by the CCRG is ultraviolet light. Prolonged exposure to ultraviolet light has been shown in laboratory animals to damage the lens and the retina, and its role in human eye disease is being investigated. The value of implants and glasses that filter ultraviolet light is also being studied.

The Guyton-Minkowski Potential
Acuity Meter

Will you see better after cataract surgery? This question is basic to all cataract surgery because there is no purpose to the operation unless it will improve your sight.

About 10 percent of patients with cataracts dense enough to impair vision have macular degeneration, also bad enough to impair vision. Ophthalmologists and their patients thus are often faced with a dilemma: Which is responsible for the poor vision, the cataract or the retina? Just as the cataract prevents the patient from looking out, it may also prevent the doctor from looking in and examining the retina to judge to what extent the cataract is impairing vision. The dilemma has been largely resolved by an ingeniously simple device called the Potential Acuity Meter (PAM), developed by two ophthalmologists at Johns Hopkins University, Dr. David L. Guyton and Dr. John S. Minkowski, and produced by Mentor O&O, Inc., of Hingham, Massachusetts. The PAM, mounted on the slit lamp, projects an eye chart, via a tiny beam of light one-quarter the diameter of a pin, through minute clear areas of the cataract, directly onto the retina. You can then read the eye chart as if the cataract were not there. This indicates your potential for vision in the eye once the cataract is removed (and it reassures you that your vision will indeed be a lot better after surgery). My own PAM arrived about a month before I wrote this chapter, and it is a remarkable instrument.

Refractive Corneal Surgery

Surgically altering the shape of the cornea is a relatively new way to correct vision after cataract surgery. Since the lens is responsible for about one-third the focusing power of the eye (the cornea is responsible for the other two-thirds), cataract surgery leaves the eye that much short of focusing ability. If at some point after cataract surgery the ability of the cornea to bend or refract light could be enhanced by surgically altering its shape, then the cornea could take over the function formerly performed by the lens. Light could be focused on the retina without an implant or contact lens. That is what refractive corneal surgery, now in its infancy, attempts to do. Several operations have been developed that involve either removing a piece of the patient's own cornea or using a piece of donor cornea and reshaping it in a machine called a cryolathe. The reshaped, more powerful cornea is then sewn back onto the eye.

All refractive corneal operations for aphakia are currently being investigated in laboratory animals and in carefully controlled human studies. The two main problems with them are delayed improvement in vision, taking up to six to twelve months for healing and good vision, and the inability to predictably correct the total focusing power a patient needs after cataract surgery. Modifications in surgical technique and cryo-lathe procedures may solve these problems in the next few years, giving patients another option besides contact lenses and implants. Children who have had congenital cataracts removed will especially benefit from refractive corneal surgery because they are not as suitable as adults for contact lenses and implants.

Lasers and Cataract Surgery

For years patients have asked, "Will my cataract be removed with a laser?" Until recently the answer was a definite no, as lasers were not used in cataract surgery. However, now the answer is a qualified yes.

Lasers have been used extensively in ophthalmology for treating glaucoma and retina trouble from diabetes, and have almost replaced two glaucoma operations, saving thousands of patients the increased risk of surgery. The argon laser commonly used in ophthalmology is only effective on pigmented tissue such as the blood in blood vessels and the pigment in the iris. The pigmented tissue absorbs the laser energy and in turn is destroyed by it. A cataract is almost unaffected by the argon laser. But a new laser, known as the Neodynium: YAG laser, developed by Professor Danielle Aron-Rosa at the Trousseau Eye Clinic in

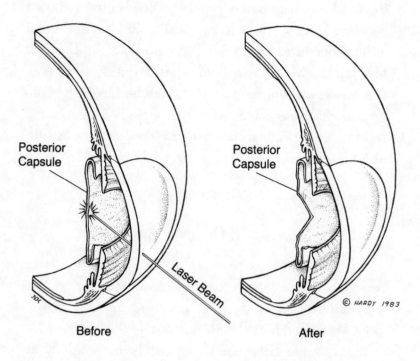

Figure 10. The YAG laser opening a cloudy posterior capsule.

Paris does not depend on pigment for its action. It uses a crystal of Yttrium Aluminum Garnet and the light is several million times brighter than that of an incandescent bulb. This new laser delivers a 500,000-watt burst of energy in a trillionth of a second! It can be focused to a minute point on the capsule of the cataract, cutting it like a tiny pair of scissors.

After extracapsular cataract surgery approximately

20 percent of patients find their posterior capsule has clouded over. A few bursts from the YAG laser can open a hole in the capsule, resulting in immediate improvement in vision (*see Figure 10*). Before the advent of the YAG laser, this capsule had to be surgically cut, and although it was a simple operation, it was still an operation and hence had some risk. YAG laser surgery can be performed painlessly and quickly at your doctor's office or in the hospital. There are only a few of these lasers in the United States, but several companies are trying to produce enough laser systems to meet a growing demand. The Neodynium-YAG laser will have a significant impact on ophthalmic surgery in the near future.

Even without these advances cataract surgery is one of the most successful of all operations. Except for the 10 percent of cataract patients who have retina trouble as well as cataracts, the chance of recovery of normal, clear vision after cataract surgery is nearly 95 percent. As advances continue this high success rate will be even higher. To the vast majority of patients it means improved eyesight, better quality of life and prevention of blindness. It is my hope that this book will help you attain these goals.

Index

Page numbers in *boldface italics* indicate illustrations.

151